Fast Facts

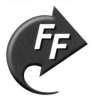

Fast Facts:
Hypertension

Third edition

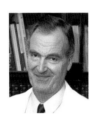

Graham A MacGregor FAHA FRCP

Professor of Cardiovascular Medicine
Department of Cardiac and Vascular Sciences
St George's Hospital Medical School
University of London
London, UK

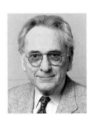

Norman M Kaplan MD

Professor of Clinical Medicine
Department of Internal Medicine
University of Texas
Southwestern Medical Center
Dallas, Texas, USA

Declaration of Independence

This book is as balanced and as practical as we can make it.
Ideas for improvements are always welcome:
feedback@fastfacts.com

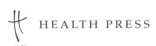

HEALTH PRESS

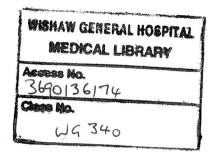
Fast Facts: Hypertension
First published 1998
Second edition 2001
Third edition April 2006

Text © 2006 Graham A Macgregor, Norman M Kaplan
© 2006 in this edition Health Press Limited
Health Press Limited, Elizabeth House, Queen Street, Abingdon,
Oxford OX14 3LN, UK
Tel: +44 (0)1235 523233
Fax: +44 (0)1235 523238

Book orders can be placed by telephone or via the website.
For regional distributors or to order via the website, please go to:
www.fastfacts.com
For telephone orders, please call 01752 202301 (UK), +44 1752 202301 (Europe),
1 800 247 6553 (USA, toll free) or +1 419 281 1802 (Americas).

Fast Facts is a trademark of Health Press Limited.

A CIP record for this title is available from the British Library.

ISBN 1-903734-60-6

MacGregor, GA (Graham)
Fast Facts: Hypertension/
Graham A Macgregor, Norman M Kaplan

Typesetting and page layout by Zed, Oxford, UK.
Printed by Fine Print (Services) Ltd, Oxford, UK.

Printed with vegetable inks on fully biodegradable and
recyclable paper manufactured from sustainable forests.

NORDIC ENVIRONMENTAL LABEL
444   001
Low emissions
during production

Low
chlorine

Sustainable
forests

Introduction

Raised blood pressure is the biggest cause of death and disability in the world. Treatment trials have uniformly demonstrated major reductions in cardiovascular disease (i.e. stroke, heart failure and heart attack). Thus, the need for more effective management of hypertension is obvious, even in developed societies such as the UK and the USA, where still today fewer than one-third of hypertensive individuals are being adequately treated. As a result, many hundreds of people are dying, or suffering unnecessarily, from strokes, heart failure and heart attacks.

Since the last edition of *Fast Facts: Hypertension* in 2001, several very important clinical trials have been published, guidelines for the effective management of high blood pressure have been modified and simplified treatment regimens have been introduced.

We hope that this new, up-to-date and concise edition will prove useful in the better management of this very common and devastating medical condition.

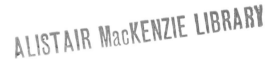

High blood pressure is the most common chronic medical condition. Approximately 30% of the adult population have an increased blood pressure, with diastolic pressure equal to or greater than 90 mmHg or systolic pressure equal to or greater than 140 mmHg. Blood pressure gradually and progressively rises with increasing age, such that raised blood pressure is seen in 20% of 20-year-olds, 40% of 40-year-olds and 60% of 60-year-olds.

Stroke and coronary heart disease

Hypertension is the most important risk factor for stroke and one of the three major risk factors for coronary heart disease (CHD). It is also the major contributory factor in over 90% of individuals who develop heart failure, as well as an important cause of accelerated renal disease.

Cardiovascular disease is responsible for just under half of all deaths and is the major cause of disability. Worldwide, raised blood pressure is responsible for more than 60% of all strokes and half of all heart disease.

Population studies. The risk of stroke or CHD is directly related to the level of blood pressure above a systolic pressure of 115 mmHg (Figure 1.1) (i.e. more than 80% of all adults). Individuals in the uppermost fifth of the blood pressure distribution have a 16-fold increase in risk of stroke compared with those in the lowest fifth. However, because there are fewer people with very high blood pressure than the much larger number with slightly elevated pressure, most strokes and CHD occur in those with only slightly elevated or 'high normal' pressure. For this reason, it is vitally important not only to treat those with high blood pressure, who individually are at greater risk, but also to develop strategies to reduce the blood pressure of the population as a whole, because this too will have a major effect on the incidence of stroke and heart disease.

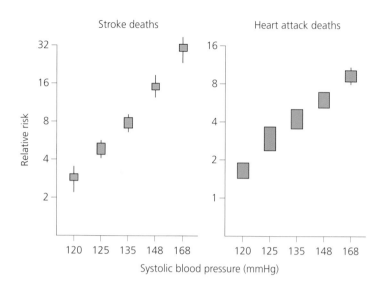

Figure 1.1 Risk of stroke or death from heart attack related to systolic blood pressure (quintiles). These data show that the risk of stroke and heart attack deaths increases throughout the range of blood pressure, starting at 115 mmHg. Note that there are insufficient numbers of people in the population with systolic blood pressure < 115 mmHg to determine whether the risk starts at even lower levels. The bars indicate 95% confidence limits; the size of the boxes is proportional to the number of events. Adapted from the Prospective Studies Collaboration, Lewington et al. 2002, with permission of Elsevier. © 2002.

Age and sex. Blood pressure – particularly systolic – increases progressively throughout adult life. Such an increase reflects a high salt intake and low potassium intake, and is not seen in unacculturated communities.

For any given blood pressure level, older people have a higher risk of death within a defined time than younger people. The highest fifth of the blood pressure distribution is associated with an annual mortality of about 3% in 45-year-olds compared with 5% at 55 years and 8% at 65 years.

Women have a lower risk of stroke or CHD than men at all levels of blood pressure until around 60 years of age, after which their risk increases to the same level as men.

Ethnic groups. Black people tend to have higher blood pressure than white people, and this is associated with a higher overall mortality, particularly from cerebrovascular disease, renal disease and heart failure. South Asian people have higher rates of stroke and CHD than white people; both CHD and diabetes are also very common.

Hypertension is common in Japan, northern China and Korea, where it is associated with a very high incidence of strokes. However, because of their previously low fat intake, these populations have, up until now, had a low incidence of CHD. Among Japanese who move to the USA and adopt a westernized diet (with less salt but more fat), the incidences of hypertension and stroke are reduced; the incidence of CHD, however, increases to the same level as that of the US population. These findings highlight the important association of salt intake with high blood pressure, and of fat intake and cholesterol with vascular disease.

Major modifiable risk factors

Hypertension interacts with a number of risk factors to determine the total risk of stroke or CHD (Table 1.1). The two major modifiable risk factors that compound with high blood pressure to increase the risk of vascular disease are smoking and blood cholesterol. Data from many prospective epidemiological studies show that these risk factors have marked additive effects with

TABLE 1.1

Major risk factors for stroke or coronary heart disease

Modifiable	Non-modifiable
Elevated blood pressure	Age
Smoking	Sex
Dyslipidemia	Ethnic origin
Diabetes or glucose intolerance	Family history
Male-pattern obesity	Previous heart attack or stroke
Lack of exercise	

hypertension (Figure 1.2). Thus a non-smoker with mild hypertension and an average cholesterol level has a much lower cardiovascular risk than someone with the same blood pressure who smokes and has elevated cholesterol. In view of the major additive interaction between these three risk factors, treatment of high blood pressure involves not only lowering the blood pressure, but also treating these other modifiable risk factors. Another important risk factor is diabetes or glucose intolerance. The number of people with diabetes is increasing rapidly as obesity becomes more common. The majority of people with diabetes are at the same risk of cardiovascular disease as those who have had a heart attack.

Defining hypertension

Within the population, blood pressure follows a normal distribution, and no clear distinction can be made between normotensive and hypertensive individuals. The risk of CHD or stroke relates directly to the blood pressure throughout the range of blood pressures, and it is not possible to establish a dividing line between a level of blood pressure that carries no risk and one that is associated with risk of cardiovascular disease. Hence, hypertension is best defined

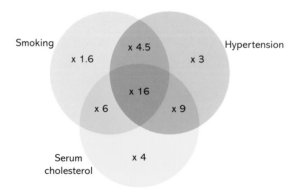

Figure 1.2 Smoking, high blood pressure and increased blood cholesterol have additive effects on the relative risk of vascular disease. Adapted from Poulter N et al. *Cardiovascular Disease and Practical Issues for Prevention.* St Albans: Caroline Black, 1993.

pragmatically – i.e. as the level above which treatment trials have shown that lowering the blood pressure is beneficial. In practice, this means either:

- a consistent diastolic blood pressure of 90 mmHg or higher, when the patient is used to the measurement of blood pressure
- a consistent systolic blood pressure of 140 mmHg or higher.

Systolic blood pressure in epidemiological studies is a better predictor of cardiovascular risk than is diastolic pressure, especially in older people. Treatment trials have historically used diastolic pressure as a treatment indicator, but nowadays treatment decisions should be based on either measurement. In addition to this pragmatic definition, hypertension has been conventionally defined according to its severity (Table 1.2), though differences between criteria have led to unnecessary confusion. The 2003 report of the US Seventh Joint National Committee on Detection, Evaluation and Treatment of High Blood Pressure (JNC VII) categorizes all levels above 120/80 mmHg and up to 140/90 mmHg as 'prehypertension', primarily to encourage acceptance of lifestyle changes that will slow down the increase in blood pressure that would otherwise occur and therefore reduce cardiovascular disease. If these measures are successful, the need for subsequent drug treatment may be delayed or avoided.

Damaging effects

Hypertension causes damage to the heart, brain and kidneys. This results either directly as a consequence of high blood pressure or the accelerated atherosclerosis that high blood pressure causes.

Direct effects of high blood pressure

Left ventricular hypertrophy. The work of the heart increases as blood pressure rises, leading to compensatory enlargement of the heart, particularly the left ventricle (left ventricular hypertrophy; LVH). In patients with LVH, there is increased risk of myocardial infarction (4-fold) and of stroke (12-fold), as well as an increased risk of arrhythmias, compared with patients who have a comparable blood pressure but no hypertrophy.

TABLE 1.2

Arbitrary definitions of hypertension in adults based on severity: British Hypertension Society (BHS-IV) and Seventh Joint National Committee (JNC VII) criteria

Adapted from BHS-IV guidelines[*,†,‡]

Category	Systolic (mmHg)		Diastolic (mmHg)
• Optimal	< 120		< 80
• Normal	< 130		< 85
• High-normal	130–139		85–89
• Grade 1 hypertension (mild)	140–159		90–99
• Grade 2 hypertension (moderate)	160–179		100–109
• Grade 3 hypertension (severe)	≥ 180		≥ 110
• Isolated systolic hypertension			
– Grade 1	140–159		< 90
– Grade 2	≥ 160		< 90

JNC VII guidelines[*,†,§]

Category	Systolic (mmHg)		Diastolic (mmHg)
• Normal	< 120	and	< 80
• Prehypertension	120–139	or	80–89
• Stage 1 hypertension	140–159	or	90–99
• Stage 2 hypertension	≥ 160	or	≥ 100

*These guidelines apply to those who are not taking antihypertensive drugs and who are not acutely ill. When systolic and diastolic blood pressures fall into different categories, the higher category should be selected to classify the individual's blood pressure status.
†Based on the average of two or more readings taken at each of two or more visits after an initial screening.
‡Adapted from Williams et al. 2004.
§Adapted from Chobanian et al. 2003.

Heart failure. With the additional load it places on the heart, raised blood pressure is now recognized as the major cause of heart failure, particularly if there is associated coronary heart disease.

Microvascular aneurysms. Charcot Bouchard aneurysms can develop in intracerebral arteries. Rupture of these aneurysms leads to intracerebral hemorrhage (Figure 1.3). Larger aneurysms in the Circle of Willis are at particular risk of rupture if there is associated high blood pressure causing either cerebral hemorrhage or subarachnoid hemorrhage.

Lacunar infarcts. High blood pressure can also lead to damage to the very small branches of the middle cerebral arteries, with the formation of lacunar infarcts, particularly in the thalamus, mid-brain and pons. The exact location determines whether these cause profound neurological damage, or have less severe consequences such as impaired memory and cognitive skills.

Renal failure. Severe hypertension in the accelerated or malignant form can lead to progressive renal damage and, ultimately, to renal failure. Non-black individuals who are not in the accelerated phase but develop renal failure are likely to have underlying renal disease. In patients with underlying renal disease, raised blood pressure can markedly accelerate the deterioration in renal function.

Aortic aneurysm and dissection are also direct consequences of raised blood pressure.

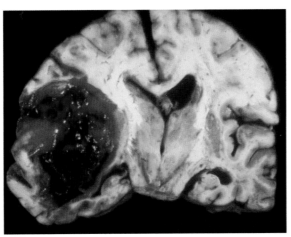

Figure 1.3
A large cerebral hemorrhage. Reproduced with permission from MacGregor GA. *Diagnostic Picture Tests in Hypertension.* London: Mosby-Wolfe, 1996.

Indirect effects of high blood pressure

Atherosclerosis. Approximately 19 out of 20 of us are developing atheroma and atheromatous plaques (Figure 1.4). The rate at which these plaques develop and their sites largely determine (in 4 out of 10 people) when we die.

High blood pressure hastens the development of the plaques and destabilizes them, making ulceration of the cap and plaque fissure much more likely. If the plaque ulcerates, platelets are attracted to the site and a thrombus forms. The higher the blood pressure, the more likely the thrombus is to become unstable and bits (emboli) are to be dislodged, causing damage further down the artery. However, if a plaque fissures, thrombus formation may spread out into and occlude the artery (Figure 1.5). Depending on which organ the artery supplies, this can lead to myocardial infarction or cerebral thrombosis.

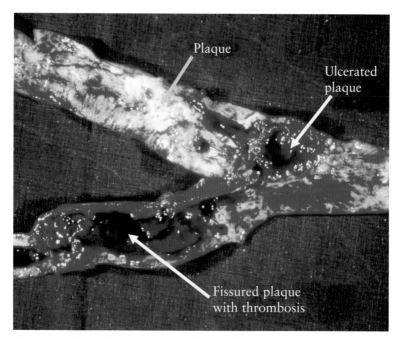

Figure 1.4 Atherosclerosis in the carotid artery bifurcation of a 45-year-old patient. Adapted with permission from MacGregor GA. *Diagnostic Picture Tests in Hypertension*. London: Mosby-Wolfe, 1996.

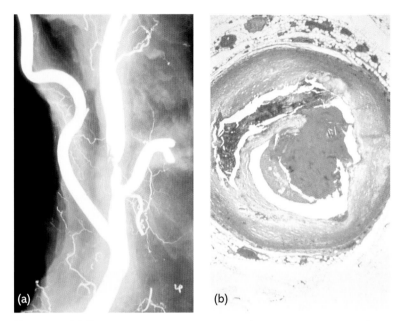

Figure 1.5 (a) Post-mortem coronary angiogram showing severe stenosis of the coronary artery. (b) Histological section across the lesion shows a ruptured plaque that has spread and caused occlusion of the lumen of the artery. This is the most common cause of death in the world. Reproduced with permission from MacGregor GA. *Diagnostic Picture Tests in Hypertension*, courtesy of Professor M Davies. London: Mosby-Wolfe, 1996.

Atherosclerosis in the peripheral vessels may lead to intermittent claudication, and may cause narrowing of renal arteries; if of a sufficient degree, it may cause high blood pressure.

High blood pressure leads to abnormalities of endothelial function, changes in arterial compliance and more turbulent flow. This turbulent flow occurs particularly at junctions of arteries, where eddy currents may form immediately adjacent to the arterial wall, causing reduction in flow and sudden changes in shear stress. These effects facilitate lipid transport into the atheromatous lesion. If the blood pressure is lowered, not only are the direct effects of high blood pressure reduced, but the rate of progression of the underlying atherosclerosis is markedly reduced and stabilization of the plaques is immediate.

Key points – the importance of hypertension

- Raised blood pressure is the major cause of cardiovascular disease in the world.
- The risks increase progressively from a systolic pressure of 115 mmHg.
- The majority of people will develop high blood pressure as they grow older.
- Blood pressure causes damage by the direct effects of the increased pressure and indirectly by markedly accelerating atherosclerosis and destabilizing plaques.
- A population strategy to lower blood pressure and gain better control of raised blood pressure would cause an immense reduction in cardiovascular disease, i.e. strokes, heart failure and heart attacks.

Key references

Burt VL, Whelton P, Roccella EJ et al. Prevalence of hypertension in the US adult population. Results from the Third National Health and Nutrition Examination Survey, 1988–1991. *Hypertension* 1995;25:305–13.

Chobanian AV, Bakris GL, Black HR et al. The seventh report of the Joint National Committee on prevention, detection, evaluation, and treatment of high blood pressure: the JNC 7 report. *JAMA* 2003;289:2560–72.

Kannel WB. Elevated systolic blood pressure as a cardiovascular risk factor. *Am J Cardiol* 2000;85:251–5.

Kaplan NM. *Kaplan's Clinical Hypertension*, 9th edn. Philadelphia: Lippincott, Williams and Wilkins, 2006.

Lawes CM, Rodgers A, Bennett DA et al. Blood pressure and cardiovascular disease in the Asia Pacific region. *J Hypertens* 2003;21:707–16.

Lewington S, Clarke R, Qizilbash N et al. Age-specific relevance of usual blood pressure to vascular mortality: a meta-analysis of individual data for one million adults in 61 prospective studies. *Lancet* 2002;360:1903–13.

Vasan RS, Beiser A, Seshadri S et al. Residual lifetime risk for developing hypertension in middle-aged women and men. The Framingham Heart Study. *JAMA* 2002;287:1003–10.

Williams B, Poulter NR, Brown MJ et al. British Hypertension Society guidelines for hypertension management 2004 (BHS-IV): summary. *BMJ* 2004;328:634–40.

Essential hypertension (primary or idiopathic), for which there is no overt cause, accounts for 95% of all cases. Of those remaining, most are due to renovascular or renal disease, or disorders of the adrenal gland. Essential hypertension – the 'silent killer' – is a progressive condition that remains asymptomatic, unless very severe. It manifests itself either in coronary artery disease or cerebrovascular disease (e.g. heart attack or stroke) without warning. Blood pressure may start to increase in childhood or even infancy. The tendency towards high blood pressure is known to run in families, but exposure to environmental factors (which cause a gradual and progressive rise in blood pressure as people age) is needed to cause the increase. The principal ones are shown in Table 2.1.

Salt intake

The most important factor that can cause a rise in blood pressure is salt intake. Evidence for this comes from six separate sources:
- epidemiological studies
- migration studies
- intervention studies
- treatment trials
- genetic studies
- animal models.

TABLE 2.1

Principal factors in the development of essential hypertension

- High salt intake
- Low potassium intake (lack of fruit and vegetables in the diet)
- Excess weight (particularly if abdominal)
- Physical inactivity
- Excessive alcohol intake (transient effect)

Epidemiological and migration studies, particularly the Intersalt study, clearly demonstrate that salt intake is related to blood pressure both between and within different communities, and is related to the rise in blood pressure with age that occurs in all countries in which salt intake is more than 6 g/day (Figure 2.1).

Intervention studies. In a study of two villages in Portugal, the inhabitants of one village were given advice to lower salt intake and were provided with processed food containing less salt, while those in the other village remained on their usual diet. At the end of the 2-year intervention period, there was a highly significant difference between the average blood pressures in the two villages, demonstrating the effect in a community of reducing salt intake.

Treatment trials. Well-controlled randomized studies, both in hypertensive and normotensive subjects, have shown that, over 1 month, a moderate reduction in salt intake (i.e. from 10–12 g/day to 5–6 g/day) causes a fall in blood pressure. These falls in blood pressure are greater in individuals with lower levels of plasma renin activity, for example, people of African descent or

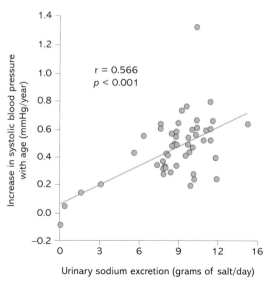

Figure 2.1 The large international Intersalt study showed that the increase in blood pressure with age in developed societies is directly related to the salt content of the diet. Reproduced from the Intersalt Cooperative Research Group 1988, with permission of BMJ Publishing Group. Copyright © 1988.

older individuals. Furthermore, a reduction in salt intake has been shown to have an additive effect to drug treatment.

Two studies – a randomized double-blind crossover study of three different salt intakes and the DASH sodium trial (also investigating three different salt intakes) – have shown a clear dose response, that is, the bigger the reduction in salt intake, the larger the fall in blood pressure.

A recent meta-analysis of all studies of 1 month or more showed highly significant falls in blood pressure in both normotensive and hypertensive individuals and a dose response to salt reduction (see pages 52–54).

A reduction in salt of 6 g/day correlates with a fall in systolic blood pressure of 7 mmHg in hypertensives and 4 mmHg in normotensives. This level of salt reduction translates into a 24% reduction in deaths due to stroke and a 20% reduction in the incidence of heart disease.

Genetic studies. Almost all currently identified single-gene defects that cause high blood pressure in humans either involve a tubular defect in the kidneys' ability to excrete sodium or an imposed restraint on the kidneys' ability to excrete sodium. Genetic causes of low blood pressure in contrast cause a defect in the kidneys' ability to reabsorb sodium.

Animal models. Hypertension in animal models is either caused or exacerbated by a high salt intake. In a study in chimpanzees (which have a 99% genetic homology with humans), a group fed a diet containing 10–15 g salt/day experienced a large increase in blood pressure within 1 year compared with a control group kept on their normal diet, which contained 0.5 g salt/day.

Recommendations. All the evidence relating salt to blood pressure, particularly the results of treatment trials and meta-analyses, shows that salt intake must be reduced worldwide from the current intake of 10–12 g/day to a much lower level. This has been arbitrarily set at an achievable target of around 5–6 g/day.

In developed countries, 75–80% of the salt consumed is hidden in foods (e.g. in processed ready meals, fast foods and restaurant/ canteen foods) and the consumer has no control over it. Another 5% of salt is naturally present in foods, which leaves, on average, 15% within the control of the consumer, either as salt added during cooking or at the table. From a population perspective, it is therefore vital that the food industry as a whole gradually reduces the amount of salt in foods.

A reduction in the salt concentration of a given food by 10–25% is undetectable by human taste receptors. As salt intake falls, the taste receptors become more sensitive and foods with lower salt concentrations taste just as salty as previously tasted foods with high salt concentrations.

In the UK, a policy aimed at reducing salt intake is now being pursued. The amount of salt in foods is gradually being reduced, with a target of 6 g/day by 2010. Many European countries are starting to follow the UK's lead. Individuals with high blood pressure have a greater need to reduce their salt intake now and need careful instructions on how to do so, given that most foods currently contain very high concentrations of salt.

Potassium intake

A high potassium intake protects against some of the effects of a high salt intake on blood pressure, and much epidemiological evidence also suggests that a high dietary potassium intake is associated with a lower blood pressure.

Studies of black people in the USA have shown that, where salt intake is similar to that of white people, the higher prevalence of increased blood pressure among black people is associated with lower potassium intake. However, most communities that consume a high level of potassium tend to eat less salt. Increases in potassium intake, either by taking potassium chloride or, preferably, by increasing fruit and vegetable consumption to at least five portions a day, have been associated with clinically important reductions in blood pressure and a reduction in the risk of strokes and heart disease.

Weight

There is a significant association between obesity and hypertension that cannot be fully accounted for by an overestimation of blood pressure arising from the use of an inappropriately sized cuff (see page 31). In clinical trials, weight loss almost always causes a fall in blood pressure.

In some obese patients, there are other metabolic disturbances resulting in elevated blood lipids (particularly triglycerides), glucose intolerance and insulin resistance. Other factors being equal, male-pattern abdominal obesity, as measured by a waist circumference > 94 cm in men and > 80 cm in women, carries a higher risk of cardiovascular disease.

The food industry is now targeting young children with very calorie-dense snacks, high in fat, sugar and salt. High salt intake leads to greater consumption of soft drinks (which can contain up to 8 teaspoons of sugar per can), and an epidemic of obesity and diabetes is inevitable unless action is taken.

Alcohol

High alcohol consumption is associated with increasing blood pressure. However, it appears that this relationship is quite transient because, if alcohol is withdrawn, there is an immediate fall in blood pressure.

It is likely that the alcohol-related rise in blood pressure results from either a direct vasoconstrictive effect or an increase in sympathetic tone as blood alcohol levels rise. High alcohol intake does not, therefore, seem to be a cause of sustained hypertension and, indeed, is not associated with an increased risk of vascular disease.

Moderate alcohol consumption (i.e. one-half to two standard drinks per day) has a protective effect on the development of atherosclerosis, as evidenced by a 30% reduction in coronary heart disease in moderate drinkers compared with non-drinkers. Nevertheless, heavy alcohol consumption causes marked elevations in blood pressure and surreptitious alcoholism can be a cause of resistant hypertension until the underlying problem is revealed.

Physical inactivity

In addition to contributing to the rapid increase in obesity in all developed countries, physical inactivity is associated with a higher incidence of hypertension. Regular aerobic activity may lower blood pressure, even without weight loss.

Family history

High blood pressure runs in families. Studies of twins have shown that inheritance accounts for 25% of the variability in blood pressure. Genetic factors play a role in the development of hypertension, particularly expressed as a diminished ability of the kidney to excrete salt. In the right environment (i.e. high salt, low potassium intake), these individuals will retain sodium and have a greater compensatory increase in the mechanisms designed to get rid of additional sodium due to their kidneys' difficulty in excreting it. Some part of this compensatory mechanism causes the rise in blood pressure, and the rise in blood pressure itself will also increase the ability of the kidneys to overcome their defect in excreting sodium.

Stress

Although the stress associated with our modern lifestyle is often claimed to be a cause of hypertension, there is little supporting evidence. However, acute stress causes an increase in blood pressure, although this is not sustained. Studies of stress reduction have shown no fall in 24-hour ambulatory blood pressure, though some patients can learn to relax during blood-pressure measurement and can reduce their blood pressure transiently in the clinic or surgery.

Secondary causes

Renal disease. Nearly all forms of intrinsic renal disease affect the kidneys' ability to excrete sodium as glomerular and tubular function is lost. This retention of sodium, often combined with inappropriately high levels of renin secretion due to damage to the arterioles leading to the glomeruli, gives rise to elevated blood pressure (Table 2.2). All forms of glomerular damage cause hypertension. Of particular note is immunoglobulin A (IgA)

TABLE 2.2

Renal disorders causing secondary hypertension

- Renovascular (atheromatous, fibromuscular hyperplasia)
- Glomerulonephritis
- Diabetic nephropathy
- Pyelonephritis
- Polycystic kidney disease
- Connective tissue disorders (e.g. scleroderma, polyarteritis nodosa, systemic lupus erythematosus)

glomerulonephritis, which causes severe hypertension with a characteristic finding of red cells in the urine.

The formation of cysts in polycystic kidney disease gradually damages the architecture of the kidney and invariably causes high blood pressure even before any deterioration in renal function.

Diabetic nephropathy is an important cause of high blood pressure. Indeed, it is likely that the blood pressure itself plays a major role in hastening the onset of the renal failure as it does in other forms of renal disease. Meticulous control of blood pressure delays the decline in renal function in diabetic and non-diabetic patients with renal disease (see Chapter 5) and prevents much of the accelerated vascular disease.

Renovascular hypertension is due to a narrowing of one or both renal arteries caused by atherosclerosis or fibromuscular hyperplasia. After renal parenchymal disease, it is the second most common cause of secondary hypertension and may account for 5% of older individuals with high blood pressure.

In younger women, particularly in those with no evidence of peripheral vascular disease, the underlying cause is more likely to be fibromuscular hyperplasia. This is a disorder of the arterial wall that gives rise to a characteristic beaded appearance of the renal artery, with narrowing and dilation.

Atheromatous renal narrowing of the artery usually occurs in older people, those who smoke and those with evidence of peripheral vascular disease. These patients usually have progressive renal impairment, and it may be difficult to control their blood pressure.

The rise in blood pressure seems to be largely due to the narrowed artery causing reduced pressure in the glomerulus. This causes an increase in renin secretion and angiotensin II production. In turn, this results in an immediate rise in blood pressure. Concomitantly, the increase in angiotensin II directly, and through increased aldosterone secretion, causes retention of sodium and water. This is seen particularly in bilateral renal artery stenosis or in renal artery stenosis when there is only one functioning kidney. Sodium retention may be of such a degree that the renin secretion is turned down and, though plasma renin activity or angiotensin II may be in the normal range, it is inappropriate for that degree of sodium retention.

Renal artery stenosis of sufficient severity can cause renal impairment and, eventually, renal failure. Renal failure may be due to multiple cholesterol emboli or thrombosis of the renal artery. Occasionally, the sodium and water retention may be of sufficient degree to cause chronic congestive heart failure or sudden left ventricular failure, a treatable cause of heart failure that is often missed. Angiotensin-converting-enzyme (ACE) inhibitors and angiotensin-receptor blockers (ARBs) may cause a reduction in renal function in those with bilateral disease, or unilateral disease if there is only one functioning kidney. Serum creatinine should be monitored if renal artery stenosis is suspected.

Primary aldosteronism. Excessive secretion of aldosterone from the adrenal gland can either result from a unilateral adenoma of the adrenal cortex (Figure 2.2) or bilateral adrenal hyperplasia. In both cases, excessive secretion of aldosterone leads to sodium and water retention with suppression of the renin–angiotensin system and a low plasma renin activity. Characteristically, patients present with high blood pressure, a mild increase in plasma sodium to 141–145 mmol/L and a reduction in plasma potassium below 3.7 mmol/L. These abnormalities in plasma potassium and sodium

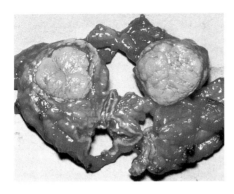

Figure 2.2 An adrenal adenoma. Reproduced with permission from MacGregor GA. *Diagnostic Picture Tests in Hypertension.* London: Mosby-Wolfe, 1996.

can be exacerbated by increased salt intake and, importantly, may be masked if patients are on a low-salt diet. It is important to distinguish patients with high aldosterone (and low renin) from those with secondary aldosteronism, in which increased renin is responsible for the increase in aldosterone (e.g. patients on a very-low-salt diet or diuretics, or those with renal artery stenosis, who will have both raised renin and aldosterone levels).

A variety of rare genetic disorders have now been described that affect aldosterone secretion or aldosterone receptors. The effect of these on blood pressure illustrates the importance of subtle changes in aldosterone, and thereby sodium retention, in the regulation of blood pressure.

Pheochromocytomas are chromaffin cell tumors that secrete excessive amounts of catecholamines, norepinephrine (noradrenaline) and epinephrine (adrenaline) (Figure 2.3).

Figure 2.3 A sectioned pheochromocytoma showing multiple hemorrhagic areas. Reproduced with permission from MacGregor GA. *Diagnostic Picture Tests in Hypertension.* London: Mosby-Wolfe, 1996.

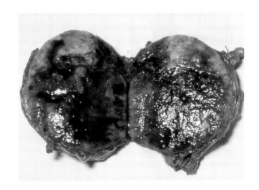

These tumors are found most commonly in the adrenal medulla, but can occur in the sympathetic ganglia (abdominal and, rarely, thoracic and those of the bladder). Release of norepinephrine and epinephrine is usually episodic, and, characteristically, these patients present with attacks of sweating, headaches, palpitations and high blood pressure. Very rarely, they may cause sustained hypertension with no symptoms.

Most of the tumors are benign, but can cause fatal hypertensive crises, particularly in pregnancy or during anesthesia. Malignant pheochromocytomas may metastasize both locally and, rarely, distally.

Improved assays for increased catecholamines in blood and urine have made the recognition of a pheochromocytoma less difficult.

Cushing's syndrome. Excessive secretion of cortisol is associated with high blood pressure, partly due to the mineralocorticoid effect of high levels of cortisol. There is also an increase in angiotensinogen from the liver, which causes an increase in angiotensin II.

Other causes

Some other causes of hypertension are shown in Table 2.3.

TABLE 2.3

Other causes of secondary hypertension

- Hormonal disturbances
  - primary hyperparathyroidism
  - hyperthyroidism
  - hypothyroidism
  - acromegaly
  - renin tumor

- Drugs (e.g. combined oral contraceptives)
- Coarctation of the aorta
- Sleep apnea
- Pregnancy-induced hypertension

Malignant hypertension

Very severe hypertension may directly damage the small renal arterioles, leading to a further increase in blood pressure. This vicious circle leads to accelerated or malignant hypertension, which can cause progressive renal failure, hypertensive encephalopathy, cerebral hemorrhage and heart failure. Before effective drug treatment became available, life expectancy was only 3–6 months.

Characteristically, patients present with severe hypertension (diastolic pressure > 130 mmHg) and hemorrhages, and/or exudates and/or papilledema in the fundi (there is no clinical distinction between these; Figure 2.4).

The condition is reversible provided the blood pressure is lowered in its early stages. In later stages, however, irreversible renal failure often develops, requiring dialysis and/or transplantation.

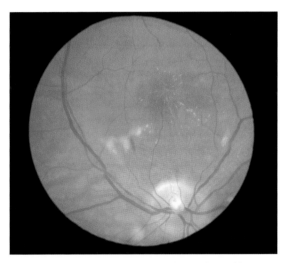

Figure 2.4 Fundus of a 32-year-old woman with accelerated hypertension, showing characteristic cotton wool spots and hard exudates. Papilledema are not present, but the striae around the disc suggest that the optic disc had been swollen in the past. The woman's blood pressure had been reduced before the photograph was taken. Reproduced with permission from MacGregor GA. *Diagnostic Picture Tests in Hypertension.* London: Mosby-Wolfe. 1996.

27

Key points – causes

- Most hypertension is of unknown cause, i.e. primary or 'essential'.
- Beyond heredity, environmental factors are responsible for hypertension, including high salt and low potassium intake, excess weight and physical inactivity.
- Alcohol in moderation is cardioprotective, but in excess (three or more standard drinks a day), it causes hypertension.
- Multiple secondary or identifiable causes of hypertension exist. Of these, renal parenchymal and renovascular disease are the most common.

Key references

Forte JG, Miguel JM, Miguel MJ et al. Salt and blood pressure: a community trial. *J Hum Hypertens* 1989;3:179–84.

He FJ, MacGregor GA. Effect of longer-term modest salt reduction on blood pressure. *Cochrane Database Syst Rev* 2005;4:CD004937. *The Cochrane Library*, issue 1. Chichester: John Wiley & Sons, 2004. www.thecochranelibrary.com

He FJ, MacGregor GA. How far should salt intake be reduced? *Hypertension* 2003;42:1093–9.

Intersalt Cooperative Research Group. Intersalt: an international study of electrolyte excretion and blood pressure. Results for 24 hour urinary sodium and potassium excretion. *BMJ* 1988;297:319–28.

Kaplan NM. The current epidemic of primary aldosteronism: causes and consequences. *J Hypertens* 2004;22: 863–9.

Luft FC. Hypertension as a complex genetic trait. *Semin Nephrol* 2002; 22:115–26.

Sawka A, Jaeschke R, Singh RJ, Young WF Jr. A comparison of biochemical tests for pheochromo-cytoma: measurement of fractionated plasma metanephrines compared with the combination of 24-hour urinary metanephrines and catecholamines. *J Clin Endocrinol Metab* 2003;88:553–8.

Whelton PK, He J, Cutler JA et al. Effects of oral potassium on blood pressure. Meta-analysis of randomized controlled clinical trials. *JAMA* 1997;277:1624–32.

The investigation of hypertension should answer four key questions.
- What is the level of blood pressure and hence the risk?
- Has the blood pressure caused any target organ damage?
- What are the other associated cardiovascular risk factors?
- Is there any underlying cause for the increase in blood pressure?

By far the most important investigation of high blood pressure is its accurate measurement, for this largely determines whether treatment will be given. This will commit patients to a lifetime of treatment – an important, and expensive, decision.

As mercury manometers are being phased out, blood pressure can be measured reliably by automatic electronic sphygmomanometers. However, many of these machines are not tested for accuracy. It is essential that every machine has been validated using a proper testing protocol (e.g. British Hypertension Society [BHS]). The BHS website, www.bhsoc.org, has a full up-to-date list.

Principles of blood pressure measurement

The conventional method for measuring blood pressure involves listening for the Korotkoff sounds (Figure 3.1). When used appropriately, these accurately reflect both systolic and diastolic pressures.

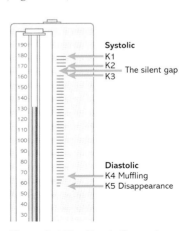

The first appearance of sounds is at systole, but occasionally in elderly people there may be a silent gap after the sounds are initially heard. It is therefore important to inflate the cuff and to feel for the disappearance of the radial

Figure 3.1 The Korotkoff sounds.

29

pulse to ensure that the cuff has been inflated above the systolic pressure before listening. When the sounds disappear, phase 5 is an accurate reflection of diastolic pressure. The muffling of sounds, phase 4, should not be taken as diastolic pressure unless the sounds continue to very low levels, as in high-output states such as pregnancy.

Technique of blood pressure measurement

- The patient should be seated comfortably with the forearm supported and the cuff placed around the arm at the level of the heart (Figure 3.2). The forearm should be slightly extended and externally rotated. Supporting the arm is important because blood pressure varies markedly depending on the position of the arm.

- Exertion, caffeine, smoking and stressful discussions should be avoided immediately before measurement.

- The cuff should be applied so that the appropriate mark is over the brachial pulse (with the brachial artery in the middle of the bladder of the sphygmomanometer), and connected to the manometer. If a mercury sphygmomanometer is used, the observer's eyes should be at the same level as the manometer.

- The cuff should be inflated slowly and steadily to a pressure 30 mmHg above that required to occlude the pulse. If it is the first time that blood pressure has been measured, it is advisable to warn the patient that there will be some discomfort as the cuff is inflated. The cuff is deflated at a rate of about 2–3 mmHg per second, and systolic and diastolic pressures recorded either automatically, or as described above.

- Blood pressures should be measured to the nearest 2 mmHg and recorded immediately.

- At the first consultation, blood pressure should be measured in both arms. A significant difference between the two arms may be a result of underestimation of blood pressure in one arm due to atheroma in the subclavian artery. In individuals with delayed or reduced femoral pulses, a leg blood pressure should be obtained.

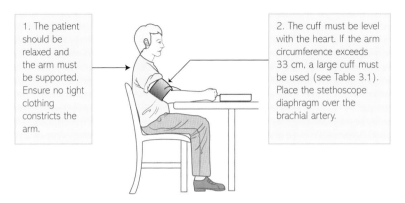

1. The patient should be relaxed and the arm must be supported. Ensure no tight clothing constricts the arm.

2. The cuff must be level with the heart. If the arm circumference exceeds 33 cm, a large cuff must be used (see Table 3.1). Place the stethoscope diaphragm over the brachial artery.

Figure 3.2 The recommended technique for measuring blood pressure with an automatic, validated, electronic machine.

Problems with blood pressure measurement

Although blood pressure measurement is a simple technique, problems can arise as a result of a number of instrumental and observer-related factors.

Sphygmomanometer-related errors. Measurement errors can arise as a result of a defective control valve, an inappropriate amount of mercury in the manometer, or a tilting or dirty mercury column. All sphygmomanometers should be serviced at least once a year.

Cuff size. Inappropriate cuff size is an important source of error in blood pressure measurement (Table 3.1). For very large arms, a bigger cuff is needed. A cuff that is too small or too narrow can cause blood pressure to be overestimated by up to 30 mmHg. Conversely, the use of too large a cuff can lead to underestimations.

TABLE 3.1

Recommended cuff sizes for blood pressure measurement

• Adults	12.5–13 cm × 23 cm
• Adults (obese)	12.5–13 cm × 35 cm
• Children > 10 years (and lean adult arms)	7.5–9 cm × 22–23.5 cm

Observer errors. Faulty technique can result in inaccurate measurements. Failure to inflate the cuff sufficiently to occlude the brachial pulse, for example, results in underestimation of systolic blood pressure. If the observer's eye is not level with the top of the mercury column, parallax errors can result.

Inaccuracy also results from a tendency to round blood pressure measurements up or down, usually to the nearest 5 or 10 mmHg (terminal digit preference). The importance of blood pressure as a predictor of survival in individuals means that it is essential to measure it as accurately as possible.

A third potential source of error is observer bias. This could lead to a borderline measurement being recorded as normal for a young healthy patient, but hypertensive for a middle-aged patient with a similar reading.

Automatic validated electronic sphygmomanometers are now increasingly being used to measure blood pressure. These machines have the great advantage of eliminating the need for auscultation (which can be tedious) and the potential for observer bias. It is also much easier to repeat blood pressure measurements, and, if required, these can be taken at a single consultation.

Mercury is potentially toxic, so mercury sphygmomanometers are gradually being phased out in most countries. It is vitally important that a standard method of blood pressure measurement is adopted (see page 30) and that a properly validated sphygmomanometer is used (see www.bhsoc.org).

Many physicians are now advising patients to buy their own monitors, so that they can measure blood pressure accurately at home. This is helpful in analysing blood pressure levels away from a clinical environment and for monitoring the efficacy of treatment. In this way, patients can take a greater part in managing their own blood pressure, with the likelihood of better control. It is important that patient leaflets are designed to give the correct information about the sort of monitors to buy. Only upper arm units should be considered. Wrist monitors, whilst technically accurate, suffer from tremendous variability depending on the position of the wrist.

Variability. The typical marked variability of blood pressure, often related to emotional or physical stress, can be best recognized by 24-hour ambulatory blood pressure monitoring (ABPM; Figure 3.3). Such variability explains the essential need for multiple readings to establish the range of blood pressure before the diagnosis of hypertension is made, except in the few patients with dangerously high levels. As ABPM equipment is not generally available, multiple readings taken at home under varying conditions with an electronic device will help to provide the information necessary to make decisions about treatment.

White-coat hypertension. Apart from the technical aspects, many other factors can affect an individual's blood pressure. For example, patients may initially be anxious and feel threatened, particularly by the doctor or other healthcare professionals, or may have large rises in blood pressure as soon as the cuff starts to inflate. Patients should be relaxed and sitting comfortably, with their arm supported, when the blood pressure is measured. Use readings only when they have become accustomed to the technique.

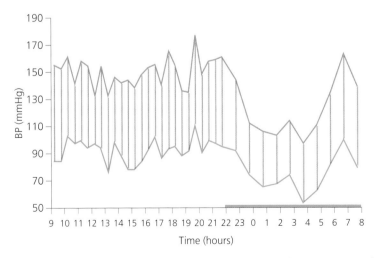

Figure 3.3 A 24-hour ambulatory blood pressure (BP) recording in a 55-year-old woman. ———————— Systolic BP; ———————— diastolic BP. Note the large fall in blood pressure during sleep (————————).

Those who continue to have a marked rise in blood pressure every time it is measured are often labeled as 'white-coat hypertensives'. Although these individuals are at less risk than those with sustained elevation, there is now evidence that this form of hypertension may carry risks and may well precede the development of more sustained blood pressure. It is helpful to perform 24-hour ABPM, as it is often found that the blood pressure is elevated initially (when the machine is applied), but soon falls and remains normal across a 24-hour period. Alternatively, patients may be encouraged to measure their blood pressure at home. This may distinguish those patients who have sustained elevation from those who have transient elevations because of the stress of entering a clinic or hospital.

Routine investigations

Any patient being considered for drug treatment for high blood pressure should undergo the following investigations.

Blood tests should be carried out on all patients (Table 3.2), and should be repeated at appropriate intervals. It is particularly important to monitor:

- plasma potassium levels if the patient is taking diuretics
- renal function, particularly if ACE inhibitors or angiotensin II antagonists have been given
- cholesterol levels (ideally fasting, with measurement of high-density lipoprotein [HDL], low-density lipoprotein [LDL] and triglycerides) as an independent risk factor for atherosclerosis
- fasting blood sugar – even small increases above average indicate a much greater risk of cardiovascular disease.

Urine tests. Urinalysis should be performed routinely (Table 3.3). In addition, 24-hour urinary sodium and potassium excretion levels are good guides to salt and potassium intake, respectively, as nearly all of the salt eaten is excreted by the kidneys with an approximate 24-hour delay. Measurement of this index of salt intake is very useful as most patients are unaware of the large amounts of salt hidden in processed foods, which account for 70–80% of our total

TABLE 3.2

Blood tests for newly diagnosed hypertensive patients

Hematocrit

- An increase in mean corpuscular volume may indicate excessive alcohol consumption

Sodium

- High (141–145 mmol/L) in patients with primary aldosteronism

Potassium

- Most common cause of hypokalemia is diuretic treatment
- Low potassium (< 3.7 mmol/L) occurs in both primary and secondary aldosteronism

Bicarbonate

- Metabolic alkalosis, with an increased plasma bicarbonate concentration, can result from either primary aldosteronism or diuretic treatment

Creatinine, urea

- A simple guide to renal function; even small increases in creatinine or urea concentration should suggest the need for further renal investigations

Fasting blood sugar

- To exclude diabetes and/or glucose intolerance

Full lipid profile (total, LDL and HDL cholesterol; triglycerides)

- An important independent risk factor for cardiovascular disease and markedly additive to the risk caused by raised blood pressure

Further tests

- Calcium: increased in primary hyperparathyroidism with an associated increase in blood pressure
- Uric acid: elevated in about 40% of hypertensive patients; particularly elevated with renal impairment or gout

HDL, high-density lipoprotein; LDL, low-density lipoprotein.

TABLE 3.3

Urine tests for newly diagnosed hypertensive patients

Test	Reason
Protein/albumin	Proteinuria/albuminuria may occur in patients with essential hypertension and underlying renal disease
Blood	If hematuria is found, red cells should be looked for in a mid-stream urine sample; it occurs in patients with malignant hypertension and glomerular diseases, but may also indicate some other underlying cause, particularly a bladder neoplasm, and this should be investigated
Sugar	Usually indicates the presence of diabetes mellitus; check fasting blood sugar

intake. Many people claim not to be using salt, but measurement of 24-hour urinary sodium will usually show salt intake is high, because of the high levels hidden in common foods (e.g. one slice of bread contains 0.5 g of salt).

A 24-hour collection is also useful to measure creatinine clearance in order to determine the glomerular filtration rate, and urinary creatinine excretion is a good guide to the completeness of the collection. If collected in acid, it can also be used for measurement of urinary catecholamines or their metabolites to exclude a pheochromocytoma. A clear explanation with printed instructions on the bottle, as well as well-trained staff, make an accurate collection easy to achieve.

Electro- and echocardiography. An electrocardiogram (ECG) should be performed in all newly diagnosed hypertensive patients and may provide evidence of left ventricular hypertrophy (LVH) or strain (Table 3.4 and Figure 3.4). It will also show evidence of previous myocardial infarction or ischemia, and is a useful record if coronary

TABLE 3.4

ECG signs of left ventricular hypertrophy

- Biphasic P wave in leads V_1 and V_2 (not specific for left ventricular hypertrophy)
- High R waves (> 12 mm) in lead aV_F
- Sum of R wave in V_5 or V_6 and S wave in V_1 > 35 mm
- ST depression and T wave inversion ('strain' pattern) in leads V_5 and V_6

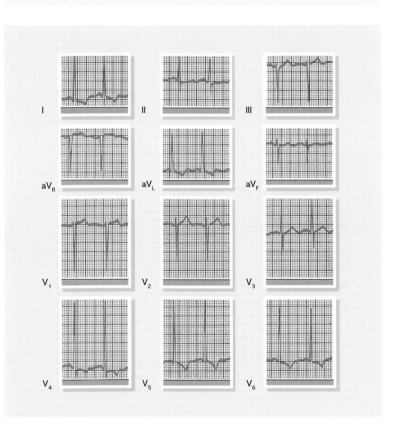

Figure 3.4 An electrocardiogram showing left ventricular hypertrophy. The patient was 61 years old and had essential hypertension. Reproduced from Hurst JW. *Atlas of the Heart.* New York: Gower Medical Publishing. Copyright © 1988.

heart disease develops. The ECG criteria for LVH are relatively insensitive; echocardiography is much more sensitive but relatively expensive for routine use. When there is evidence of LVH, the risk associated with a given blood pressure is greatly increased. Monitoring either the ECG or echocardiograms is useful to show a reduction in left ventricular mass with treatment.

24-hour ambulatory blood pressure monitoring. Used with care, ABPM devices can provide accurate profiles of blood pressure. These profiles can:
- help the diagnosis of white-coat hypertension (see pages 33–4)
- assess borderline hypertension
- evaluate symptoms that may be related to drug treatment (e.g. hypotensive episodes in the elderly).

However, the major problem with ambulatory assessment is that such measurements have not been used in outcome trials and are therefore not a clear guide to treatment. Drug treatment decisions remain based on conventional clinic measurements.

Home blood pressure recordings can fulfill a useful role, and have the advantage that patients can monitor their own blood pressure over a given period. This is not only helpful when determining indications for treatment, but also for monitoring treatment. Again, home blood pressure levels will be lower than clinic blood pressure levels, and it is difficult to determine what levels should be achieved as there are no trials that have employed either 24-hour ABPM or home blood pressure monitoring to assess the long-term benefits of treatment. Nevertheless, it is likely that both of these methods will be better predictors of cardiovascular risk than clinic pressures.

Once the appropriate trials have been done, it is likely that these will largely replace the current reliability on the small number of, often inaccurate, clinic blood pressures. Blood pressure thresholds for ABPM and home blood pressure monitoring are on average approximately 10/5 mmHg lower than clinic blood pressures, but this varies from one person to another and cannot be used to predict a difference in an individual.

Other investigations. In patients with a history or other features suggestive of a secondary cause, or those in whom there is difficulty controlling blood pressure, further investigations should be performed, and the patient should be referred to a hypertension specialist.

Renal and/or abdominal ultrasound may reveal unsuspected pathology, such as large adrenal tumors or a difference in size between the two kidneys, that may suggest renal artery stenosis (this is, however, a poor man's guide to renal artery stenosis which by no means excludes it). Renal ultrasound is very reliable for the diagnosis of polycystic kidney disease, an important cause of hypertension and renal failure.

Renal artery duplex sonography, if performed carefully by an experienced technician or radiologist, may provide adequate screening for significant renal artery stenosis.

Isotopic renography after a single oral dose of captopril has been found to be a reasonably accurate screening test for renovascular hypertension.

Magnetic resonance angiography, with a high-resolution scanner, is probably the best screening test for renal artery stenosis. However, it is still not 100% reliable and may give both false-positive and false-negative results.

Key points – investigation

- Blood pressure should be measured carefully.
- Increasingly, home and ambulatory measurements are being used to overcome the 'white-coat' effect.
- Routine testing is limited to urine analysis, blood tests (glucose, creatinine and electrolytes), lipid profile and an electrocardiogram.
- Additional investigation may be needed to determine secondary causes.
- Always consider rare but important (to the individual) secondary causes.

Renal angiography, in skilled hands, is a relatively simple, day-case procedure that provides clear pictures of the renal arteries (Figure 3.5). When digital subtraction is used, only very small amounts of dye need to be injected. Nevertheless, in patients with severe vascular disease, there is always a small risk of dislodging atheromatous fragments or of a deterioration in renal function with the dye. In renal failure, the injection of carbon dioxide instead of iodine dye can help to avoid any deterioration in renal function.

Hormonal measurements. Circulating hormone concentrations, such as plasma aldosterone and plasma renin activity, should be measured when there is a suggestion of primary aldosteronism. For patients in whom pheochromocytoma may be suspected, plasma catecholamines or metabolites and/or 24-hour catecholamines and metabolites should be measured.

CT scanning and MRI are used particularly for the assessment of adrenal causes of hypertension to localize both adrenal adenomas and pheochromocytomas.

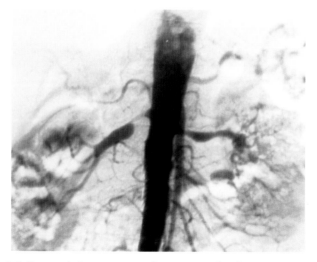

Figure 3.5 Characteristic appearance of severe vascular disease in a 60-year-old man, showing severe stenosis of the origin of the right renal artery and of the left with a post-stenotic dilation and a further constriction on the left in the middle of the renal artery. Reproduced with permission from MacGregor GA. *Diagnostic Picture Tests in Hypertension.* London: Mosby-Wolfe, 1996.

Key references

British Hypertension Society (information on blood pressure measurement and validated blood pressure monitor lists). www.bhsoc.org

Hond ED, Celis H, Fagard R et al. Self-measured versus ambulatory blood pressure in the diagnosis of hypertension. *J Hypertens* 2003;21: 717–22.

Kario K, Pickering TG, Matsuo T et al. Stroke prognosis and abnormal nocturnal blood pressure falls in older hypertensives. *Hypertension* 2001;38:852–7.

MacGregor GA. *Diagnostic Picture Tests in Hypertension*. London: Mosby-Wolfe, 1996.

Marfella R, Gualdiero P, Siniscalchi M et al. Morning blood pressure peak, QT intervals, and sympathetic activity in hypertensive patients. *Hypertension* 2003;41:237–43.

Pickering T. Recommendations for the use of home (self) and ambulatory blood pressure monitoring. American Society of Hypertension Ad Hoc Panel. *Am J Hypertens* 1996;9:1–11.

Reeves RA. The rational clinical examination. Does this patient have hypertension? How to measure blood pressure. *JAMA* 1995;273:1211–18.

Verdecchia P, O'Brien E, Pickering T et al. When can the practicing physician suspect white coat hypertension? Statement from the Working Group on Blood Pressure Monitoring of the European Society of Hypertension. *Am J Hypertens* 2003;16:87–91.

Verdecchia P, Procellati C, Schillaci G et al. Ambulatory blood pressure. An independent predictor of prognosis in essential hypertension. *Hypertension* 1994;24:793–801.

Zachariah PK, Sheps SG, Smith RL. Defining the roles of home and ambulatory monitoring. *Diagnosis* 1988;10:39–50.

The beneficial effects of using drugs to lower blood pressure are now well established. However, some of the pharmacological treatments for hypertension may have side effects. It is vital that patients are treated only if there is trial evidence which shows that treatment will be beneficial, and that the individual continues to feel completely well. It is highly unlikely that an asymptomatic patient with mild hypertension will remain on therapy that causes bothersome side effects.

Evidence from clinical trials

Severe hypertension. As soon as effective blood-pressure-lowering drugs became available in the late 1950s and early 1960s, it was clear that patients with malignant hypertension benefited from a fall in blood pressure.

The first well-controlled trial in severe hypertension, undertaken in the late 1960s – the Veterans' Study of men with a diastolic pressure between 115 and 129 mmHg randomized either to active treatment or to placebo – showed a major reduction in stroke and heart failure in little over 1 year.

Mild-to-moderate hypertension. Over the past 20 years numerous trials of antihypertensive drug therapy have shown overall reductions in the incidence of stroke by 35–40%, heart attacks by 20–25% and heart failure by more than 50%. These effects were first documented in trials using diuretics, and more recently with angiotensin-converting-enzyme (ACE) inhibitors and calcium-channel blockers.

High doses of diuretics (e.g. 100 mg hydrochlorothiazide or 10 mg bendroflumethiazide) frequently used in the 1970s and 1980s did not protect against heart attack, whereas the lower doses equivalent to 12.5–25 mg hydrochlorothiazide are cardioprotective.

Comparative treatment studies. A number of studies have compared the efficacy of different drugs. Overall, the four major classes of drugs used to treat hypertension – diuretics, calcium antagonists, ACE inhibitors and angiotensin-receptor blockers (ARBs) – all seem to be effective in reducing strokes and heart attacks.

The LIFE study (the Losartan Intervention For Endpoint reduction in hypertension study), 2002, was a well-controlled study of blood-pressure control that compared losartan (an ARB) plus a diuretic, with atenolol (a β-blocker) plus a diuretic. The two groups were equally balanced for blood pressure throughout the trial, but the atenolol group demonstrated a smaller reduction in strokes (25%) (Figure 4.1), left ventricular hypertrophy and new-onset diabetes (25%) compared with the losartan group.

The VALUE study (the Valsartan Antihypertensive Long-term Use Evaluation study), 2004, compared valsartan (an ARB) with amlodipine (a calcium antagonist). Amlodipine was slightly more effective than valsartan in preventing both strokes and heart attacks. There was a slightly lower blood pressure in the amlodipine-treated group compared with subjects receiving valsartan, which may have accounted for some of this difference.

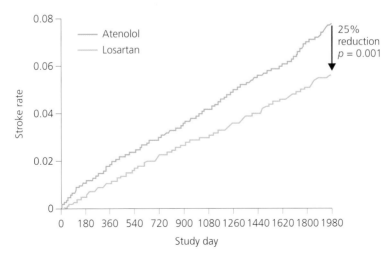

Figure 4.1 Results of the LIFE study. Patients receiving the β-blocker atenolol had significantly more strokes than patients receiving the ARB losartan.

ALLHAT (the Antihypertensive and Lipid-Lowering treatment to prevent Heart Attack Trial), 2002, compared treatment with four different drug classes: a diuretic, chlorthalidone; a calcium antagonist, amlodipine; an ACE inhibitor, lisinopril; and an α-blocker, doxazosin. The doxazosin arm was stopped early in the trial owing to an increase in apparent heart failure and less effective control of blood pressure. The amlodipine and chlorthalidone groups had almost identical results, whereas the lisinopril group experienced a higher incidence of strokes, thought to be associated with higher blood pressure. This is unsurprising given that many of the participants were black, an ethnic group in which lisinopril is known to be less effective. In contrast, a study from Australia showed than an ACE inhibitor was as effective as diuretics in reducing strokes.

ASCOT (the Anglo-Scandinavian Cardiac Outcomes Trial), 2005, compared two treatment regimens: amlodipine (a calcium antagonist) plus, if required, perindopril (an ACE inhibitor), against atenolol (a β-blocker) plus, if required, bendroflumethiazide (a diuretic) with potassium (K+). The patients recruited were aged between 40 and 70 years. As well as hypertension, all had at least three other risk factors for cardiovascular events. The strength of the trial was that primary care physicians enrolled over 50% of the study population. Treatment was intended to continue for 5 years, or until 1150 primary events (non-fatal MI, fatal CHD) occurred. The trial was stopped prematurely (after 4 years) because of a higher mortality in the atenolol ± bendroflumethiazide K+ group. The trial demonstrated that the amlodipine ± perindopril group reduced the primary endpoints, non-fatal MI or death from CHD, by 10% (not statistically significant). For most of the secondary endpoints, the amlodipine ± perindopril group had statistically significant reductions in risk – a greater reduction in strokes (by 23%), a lower cardiovascular mortality (by 24%) and a lower over-all mortality (by 11%) than the atenolol ± bendroflumethiazide K+ group (Table 4.1, Figure 4.2). Overall, the amlodipine ± perindopril group had a lower systolic blood pressure (by 2.7 mmHg), which was statistically significant. However, this difference in overall blood pressure is unlikely to account for all of the differences in outcome. Furthermore, fewer patients developed new-onset diabetes (a tertiary endpoint) in the amlodipine ± perindopril group (a 30% difference).

TABLE 4.1

ASCOT results: reduction (% difference) in primary and secondary endpoints for amlodipine ± perindopril compared with atenolol ± bendroflumethiazide K+

Endpoint	Difference	p value
Non-fatal MI, fatal CHD	10%	0.105
Fatal and non-fatal stroke	23%	< 0.001
Cardiovascular mortality	24%	< 0.01
Fatal and non-fatal heart failure	16%	0.126
All-cause mortality	11%	< 0.05
New-onset diabetes mellitus*	30%	< 0.0001

*Tertiary endpoint; CHD, coronary heart disease; MI, myocardial infarction.
Adapted from Dahlof et al. 2005, with permission of Elsevier. Copyright © 2005.

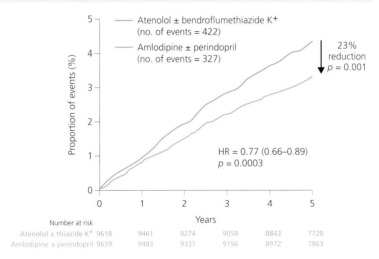

Figure 4.2 Results of the ASCOT study. Patients receiving amlodipine ± perindopril had significantly fewer strokes than patients receiving atenolol ± bendroflumethiazide K+. HR, hazard ratio. Adapted from Dahlof et al. 2005, with permission of Elsevier. Copyright © 2005.

Meta-analyses of the randomized trials described above have been conducted, although not as yet including the ASCOT study.

β-blocker regimens. Two recent meta-analyses of atenolol and other β-blockers showed that they have less effect than other drugs. A meta-analysis carried out by the National Institute for Clinical Excellence in the UK showed a clear increase in new-onset diabetes in those treated with a β-blocker and diuretic compared with other regimens. The results indicate that approximately 1 in 8 individuals would develop diabetes over a 30-year period if they were given a β-blocker regimen compared with a regimen that did not contain a β-blocker. For this and other reasons, β-blockers are no longer indicated as first-line treatment for high blood pressure unless there are specific indications such as angina, post-myocardial infarction or heart failure. It has been suggested that β-blockers may not lower central aortic pressure to the same extent as brachial artery pressure, which could possibly explain the higher incidence of strokes and heart failure in individuals receiving these drugs.

Blood pressure control. Meta-analyses have clearly demonstrated that a 5–6 mmHg reduction in blood pressure, which is relatively small compared with that seen in clinical practice, causes a 30–40% reduction in stroke, a 20–25% reduction in coronary heart disease and a 50% reduction in heart failure. In other words, most of the risk of stroke, heart failure and heart attack attributable to blood pressure seems to be reversed after only a few years of treatment with drugs that lower blood pressure.

The benefits shown in these studies are clearly related to the reduction in blood pressure and – apart from the β-blocker trials – not the treatment given. In conclusion, the control of blood pressure is far more important than the individual drugs given.

Older individuals (over 60 years of age). Historically, physicians have felt that treatment may not confer such great benefits in older individuals because of stiffening of the arteries. Numerous trials in older people have shown that the opposite is true, particularly in the short term, with significant reductions in stroke, heart attack and heart failure (Figure 4.3). This particularly applies to people with

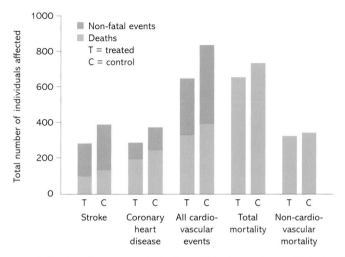

Figure 4.3 Results of a meta-analysis of 15 693 older patients with isolated systolic hypertension enrolled in eight trials of antihypertensive drug therapy. Average blood pressure at entry was 174/83 mmHg. After a median follow-up of 3.8 years, the mean difference in blood pressure between treated (T) and control (C) groups was 10.4/4.1 mmHg. Reproduced from Staessen et al. 2000, with permission of Elsevier. Copyright © 2000.

isolated systolic hypertension, for whom the risk is greater than those with combined hypertension, but the treatment benefits just as great.

There is no evidence of any reduction in benefit with increasing age, although few of the trials included participants over 80 years of age. Nevertheless, it seems prudent to treat patients over 80 years old who have severe hypertension or target organ damage, particularly as there is likely to be a major reduction in the risk of heart failure and stroke, two major causes of morbidity.

Individuals with stroke or CHD. Several trials have now demonstrated that treatment for blood-pressure control in individuals who have already had a stroke, or manifestation of early heart disease, is very worthwhile. The PROGRESS study (the Perindopril Protection against Recurrent Stroke Study) showed that the combination of an ACE inhibitor and a diuretic was effective in reducing strokes independent of the starting blood pressure level.

47

Blood pressure thresholds for treatment

Based on the above and other carefully controlled trials, several expert committees throughout the world – including the US Joint National Committee on Prevention, Detection, Evaluation and Treatment of High Blood Pressure (JNC VII), the British Hypertension Society (BHS) and the World Health Organization/ International Society of Hypertension (WHO-ISH) – have published management guidelines for the treatment of hypertension.

While there are some small differences between these guidelines, there is almost unanimous agreement on the following recommendations.

- Drug treatment should be considered if diastolic pressure is consistently above 90 mmHg and/or systolic pressure is greater than 140 mmHg after reasonable periods of observation on non-pharmacological treatment. The 2004 BHS guidelines suggest that non-pharmacological treatment should be tried first in those whose diastolic blood pressure is in the range 90–99 mmHg or whose systolic blood pressure is in the range 140–159 mmHg. Drug treatment is indicated only if there is target organ damage or evidence of established cardiovascular disease, diabetes or a 10-year cardiovascular disease risk of greater than 20%. All guidelines agree that individuals whose systolic blood pressure is greater than 160 mmHg and/or diastolic pressure is greater than 100 mmHg should be treated at any age irrespective of cardiovascular disease risk. It is important to remember that isolated systolic hypertension should be treated in an identical fashion.
- The aim of treatment should be to reduce diastolic pressure to below 85 mmHg, and systolic pressure to less than 140 mmHg. A lower target pressure may be appropriate for some elderly patients with systolic levels that are not reduced despite multiple medications, whilst a lower target of 130/80 mmHg should be achieved in patients with diabetes or renal impairment.
- Other major cardiovascular risk factors must also be treated in all patients by lifestyle changes, diet or drugs (i.e. stopping smoking, lowering cholesterol and controlling diabetes).

Key points – when to treat

- The treatment of hypertension has been shown to reduce the risks of heart attack, stroke, heart failure and renal failure.
- Patients with usual blood pressure above 140/90 mmHg should be given advice on lifestyle and considered for drug therapy.
- All major classes of drugs have been found to reduce morbidity and mortality, but recent evidence suggests that β-blockers should be avoided unless there is evidence of ischemic heart disease or heart failure.
- Older individuals (over 60 years old) obtain a relatively greater degree of protection over a short interval than younger patients.

The paradox of age

In developed countries, blood pressure increases with age, as does the risk of a cardiovascular event. A person at the age of 75 years, for example, who has a blood pressure of 160/100 mmHg, has a much greater chance of having a stroke during the next 5 years than a 35-year-old with the same blood pressure. This suggests that it is much more worthwhile to treat an elderly patient than a younger patient, as the benefits within that time period will be greater in the elderly patient. However, while events may be prevented, increases in life expectancy in the elderly will be small, whereas it is likely that treatment of high blood pressure in younger patients would increase life expectancy substantially.

Key references

ALLHAT Collaborative Research Group. Major outcomes in high-risk hypertensive patients randomized to angiotensin-converting enzyme inhibitor or calcium channel blocker vs diuretic: the Antihypertensive and Lipid-Lowering Treatment to Prevent Heart Attack Trial (ALLHAT). *JAMA* 2002;288: 2981–97.

Carlberg B, Samuelsson O, Lindholm LH. Atenolol in hypertension: is it a wise choice? *Lancet* 2004;364:1684–9.

Chalmers J, Todd A, Chapman N et al. International Society of Hypertension (ISH): statement on blood pressure lowering and stroke prevention. *J Hypertens* 2003;21: 651–63.

Chobanian AV, Bakris GL, Black HR et al. The seventh report of the Joint National Committee on Prevention, Detection, Evaluation and Treatment of High Blood Pressure: the JNC 7 report. *JAMA* 2003;289:2560–72.

Dahlof B, Devereux RB, Kjeldsen SE et al. Cardiovascular morbidity and mortality in the Losartan Intervention for Endpoint reduction in hypertension study (LIFE): a randomised trial against atenolol. *Lancet* 2002;359:995–1003.

Dahlof B, Sever PS, Poulter NR et al. Prevention of cardiovascular events with an antihypertensive regimen of amlodipine adding perindopril as required versus atenolol adding bendroflumethiazide as required, in the Anglo-Scandinavian Cardiac Outcomes Trial-Blood Pressure Lowering Arm (ASCOT-BPLA): a multicentre randomised controlled trial. *Lancet* 2005;366:895–906.

Julius S, Kjeldsen SE, Weber M et al. Outcomes in hypertensive patients at high cardiovascular risk treated with regimens based on valsartan or amlodipine: the VALUE randomised trial. *Lancet* 2004;363:2022–31.

Lindholm LH, Carlberg B, Samuelsson O. Should beta-blockers remain first choice in the treatment of primary hypertension? A meta-analysis. *Lancet* 2005; 366:1545–53.

MRC Working Party. Medical Research Council trial of treatment of hypertension in older adults: principal results. *BMJ* 1992;304:405–12.

Murray CJL, Lauer JA, Hutubessy RCW et al. Effectiveness and costs of interventions to lower systolic blood pressure and cholesterol: a global and regional analysis on reduction of cardiovascular-disease risk. *Lancet* 2003;361:717–25.

Neal B, MacMahon S, Chapman N et al. Effects of ACE inhibitors, calcium antagonists, and other blood-pressure-lowering drugs: results of prospectively designed overviews of randomised trials. *Lancet* 2000;356:1955–64.

PROGRESS Collaborative Group. Randomised trial of a perindopril-based blood-pressure-lowering regimen among 6105 individuals with previous stroke or transient ischaemic attack. *Lancet* 2001;358: 1033–41.

Sever PS, Dahlof B, Poulter NR et al. Prevention of coronary and stroke events with atorvastatin in hypertensive patients who have average or lower-than-average cholesterol concentrations, in the ASCOT-LLA: a multicentre randomised controlled trial. *Lancet* 2003;361:1149–58.

Staessen JA, Gasowski J, Wang JG et al. Risks of untreated isolated systolic hypertension in the elderly: meta-analysis of outcome trials. *Lancet* 2000;355:865–72.

Whitworth JA. 2003 WHO/ISH statement on management of hypertension. *J Hypertens* 2003;21: 1983–92.

Williams B, Poulter NR, Brown MJ et al. Guidelines for management of hypertension: report of the fourth working party of the British Hypertension Society, 2004-BHS IV. *J Hum Hypertens* 2004;18:139–85.

Zanchetti A, Hansson L, Clement D et al. Benefits and risks of more intensive blood pressure lowering in hypertensive patients of the HOT study with different risk profiles: does a J-shaped curve exist in smokers? *J Hypertens* 2003;21: 797–804.

The overall aim when treating individuals with consistently raised blood pressure is to lower their blood pressure and maintain this for the rest of their life, while keeping them feeling completely well. Given the modern therapeutic approach to high blood pressure, with both non-pharmacological advice and the large range of drugs available, it is possible to achieve this aim for the majority of people.

All individuals should be properly assessed for sustained hypertension and overt secondary causes (see pages 22–26). In addition, all patients, regardless of blood pressure level, should be given non-pharmacological advice, and attention should be paid to other cardiovascular risk factors (see pages 9–10).

Non-pharmacological measures

Several well-controlled trials have shown that non-pharmacological measures can be very effective in lowering blood pressure. However, many health professionals do not explain properly to patients and their families how to change their diet and lifestyle. Non-pharmacological measures, which have a markedly additive effect to drug therapy, include those shown in Table 5.1.

It is very important to give simple, straightforward advice to patients and to combine all of the measures detailed below into a package that patients and relatives can easily understand. As the advice is pertinent to the entire population, it is a good idea for the whole family to adopt beneficial lifestyle changes. High blood pressure and atherosclerosis are largely dietary diseases; by changing their diet, individuals can considerably modify their risk of developing vascular disease and slow down its progression.

Reducing salt intake

Considering the difficulty of achieving significant weight loss, reducing salt intake may be the most effective non-pharmacological way of lowering blood pressure (Figures 5.1 and 5.2).

TABLE 5.1

Lifestyle changes recommended for people with high blood pressure

To lower blood pressure

Reduce salt intake to < 5–6 g/day (sodium, 2.0–2.4 g/day)

Increase potassium intake (at least 5 portions/day of fruit and vegetables)

If overweight, lose weight

Limit alcohol intake to no more than 0.5–2 units/day

Increase physical activity

To reduce vascular risk

Stop smoking

Decrease saturated fat and cholesterol intake

Increase fruit and vegetable consumption (potassium, fiber)

Control blood sugar levels if diabetic

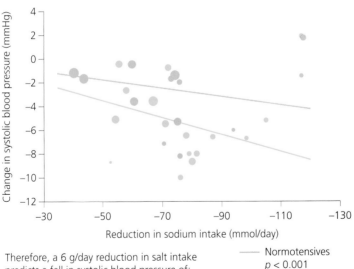

Therefore, a 6 g/day reduction in salt intake predicts a fall in systolic blood pressure of:
- 7 mmHg in hypertensives ($p < 0.001$)
- 4 mmHg in normotensives ($p < 0.01$)

—— Normotensives
$p < 0.001$

—— Hypertensives
$p < 0.001$

Figure 5.1 Meta-analysis of salt restriction studies of 1 month or more. For each study, the size of the dot is proportional to the number of participants. 50 mmol sodium = 3 g salt. Modified from He and MacGregor 2003, with permission of Lippincott Williams & Wilkins. Copyright © 2003.

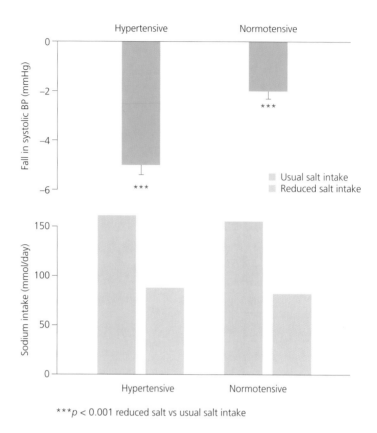

***p < 0.001 reduced salt vs usual salt intake

Figure 5.2 Meta-analysis of salt restriction studies of 1 month or more, showing that a reduction in salt intake of 5 g/day (50 mmol sodium = 3 g salt) results in significant falls in blood pressure in both hypertensive and normotensive individuals. Modified from He and MacGregor 2003, with permission of Lippincott Williams & Wilkins. Copyright © 2003.

Well-controlled clinical trials have demonstrated that reducing daily salt intake from 10–12 g/day to 5–6 g/day is as effective as single-drug therapy and, in particular, appears to have an effect similar to that of a thiazide diuretic. A meta-analysis of studies has confirmed these results and, as with diuretics, salt restriction appears to be particularly effective for older individuals, black people and those receiving drug treatment, particularly if combined with agents that inhibit or block the renin–angiotensin system.

Assessment. It is important to assess salt intake, and patients should, as part of the routine assessment of high blood pressure, have a 24-hour urine collection for measurement of sodium and potassium excretion. This will accurately reflect the patient's consumption of salt and potassium on the previous day. It is also important to repeat this test to ensure compliance and, in those with little or no dietary reduction in salt intake, to determine the reason for non-compliance.

Advising patients. There are problems with reducing salt intake. First, physicians do not give adequate instructions to patients and the person in the household who is responsible for cooking about how to cut down on salt (Table 5.2). Second, with the increasing consumption of processed and ready-prepared food, 70–80% of many patients' salt intake now comes from hidden salt in food (e.g. processed, ready-prepared, fast food, and canteen and restaurant meals). This means that patients may well stop adding

TABLE 5.2

Cutting down on salt: advice for patients

- Do not add salt to food at the table
- Do not add salt or 'flavor enhancers' made from salt (e.g. stock cubes, soy sauce) when preparing food or during cooking
- Avoid processed foods that have a high salt content. Look at the label and eat only if the sodium content is less than 200 mg/100 g (0.2 g/100 g). High-salt foods include:
  - processed meat products, cheese
  - soups
  - many instant foods
  - bread
  - some cereals
  - many ready-prepared meals
- Avoid most take-away and fast foods
- Ask for restaurant meals to be cooked with less salt

salt to their food, but there is little reduction in salt intake because of their high consumption of processed food.

Patients who have a high salt intake will initially find that food without salt will taste bland. After 3 or 4 weeks, however, the salt taste receptors become much more sensitive so that a lower salt concentration will cause the same stimulation. Indeed, most patients find that, once they are used to a low salt intake, highly salted food is unpleasant and they much prefer food without salt. Patients can be advised to use other ingredients to flavor meals, such as herbs, spices, garlic, ginger, lemon juice and chilli. Patients who are addicted to salt and have to add chemicals to their food should be advised to use a mineral salt (i.e. a mixture of potassium chloride and sodium chloride) rather than salt. It is also important to warn patients to watch out for hidden salt present in stock cubes, gravy browning, soy sauce etc.

Food labels. The food labeling system in some countries may confuse consumers. The salt content of processed foods stated in milligrams of sodium per 100 g is, for most people, meaningless. However, insight can be gained by relating the concentration of sodium to that of sea water. Atlantic sea water contains 1.0 g (1000 mg) sodium per 100 g, and this can serve as a benchmark for comparing against food labels. For instance, most bread contains 0.4–0.8 g (400–800 mg) of sodium per 100 g and so the salt concentration is between 40 and 80% that of sea water. This makes it much easier for patients to appreciate which foods contain a lot of salt, and thus be motivated to avoid them.

In the USA, food labels indicate the milligrams of sodium in a 'usual' portion of the food. Foods containing more than 300 mg per portion should be avoided. In the UK, a new label is being introduced to give the amount of salt (in grams) per serving (weight in grams) accompanied by the recommended maximum intake of salt for an adult (i.e. less than 6 g/day).

To convert sodium to salt, multiply sodium by 2.5 (e.g. 300 mg sodium = 2.5 × 300 mg salt = 0.75 g salt). Patients should aim to keep their salt intake below 6 g/day (sodium, 2.4 g/day).

Increasing potassium intake

Increasing potassium intake also lowers blood pressure. This has mostly been done in double-blind studies with potassium chloride, but more recently by increasing fruit and vegetable consumption to at least five portions per day. Patients should, therefore, be advised to eat more fresh fruit, vegetables and fish to increase their potassium intake (ideally 7–10 g/day); potassium supplements are not indicated. This move towards a more vegetarian diet has the advantage not only of increasing potassium intake, but of being low in salt and saturated fat, and high in fiber. Mineral salts that contain a mixture of potassium chloride and sodium chloride can be used if patients find it is essential to add some form of salt to their food.

Obesity and weight reduction

Many patients with high blood pressure are overweight, and it has been shown that if obese patients lose weight, there is an associated fall in blood pressure. All hypertensive patients who are overweight should therefore be encouraged to lose weight. Weight reduction is particularly effective if combined with salt restriction and an increase in fruit and vegetable consumption. Increased physical activity is almost always necessary to achieve and maintain weight loss.

Reduction of alcohol intake

There is strong epidemiological evidence of a relationship between blood pressure and alcohol. The effect is, however, short term, and a moderate intake of alcohol has protective cardiovascular effects. Patients should therefore be advised to limit their alcohol intake to a maximum of 14–21 units per week in men and 7–14 units per week in women. One unit is equivalent to approximately 10 g alcohol, which is equivalent to two-thirds of a pint of beer, a glass of wine or a standard measure of spirits. JNC VII recommends 'no more than 1 oz ethanol (e.g. 24 fluid oz beer, 10 fluid oz wine or 3 fluid oz 80-proof whisky) per day for men, or $1/_2$ fluid oz ethanol per day for women'. Physicians should be aware, however, that surreptitious alcoholism can be an important cause of resistant hypertension.

Physical activity

Regular physical activity (i.e. 30 minutes of aerobic exercise three to five times a week) may reduce blood pressure. Clearly, patients who are unfit should start with a low level of exercise – dynamic, such as walking, rather than static – and increase gradually. There is also evidence that exercise increases HDL cholesterol and that patients feel better when they are fitter. More intensive physical activity will help to achieve weight loss.

Other methods of reducing blood pressure

Many claims have been made about other dietary changes that may affect blood pressure, such as increasing calcium intake, but there is no controlled evidence to support these claims. Relaxation has also been claimed to lower blood pressure, but this appears to be due to a physiological reflex whereby blood pressure falls when muscles are relaxed (e.g. during sleep). Though patients can learn to lower their blood pressure while it is being measured, by relaxing more than the control group, 24-hour ambulatory monitoring has, disappointingly, shown no fall in blood pressure.

Smoking. It is of vital importance that other cardiovascular risk factors, such as smoking, are addressed when treating high blood pressure. Although each cigarette raises blood pressure transiently, smoking has no long-term effect on blood pressure. However, it is a very powerful risk factor for coronary heart disease (CHD), thrombotic stroke and peripheral vascular disease. This risk is markedly increased if associated with high blood pressure and raised cholesterol. All patients with high blood pressure *must* stop smoking – the risks should be made absolutely clear.

Fat intake. High LDL cholesterol and low HDL cholesterol increase the risk of vascular disease, particularly if blood pressure is also raised; smoking increases this further. It is vital when lowering blood pressure also to lower cholesterol, regardless of the starting level. Patients should reduce their consumption of saturated fats and not eat excessive amounts of cholesterol (Table 5.3).

TABLE 5.3

Reducing fat intake: advice for patients

- Reduce consumption of dairy products other than fully skimmed milk and low-fat cheeses
- Reduce red meat consumption and avoid red meat products that are also very high in salt
- Avoid baked products with fat (e.g. croissants)
- Avoid coconut and palm oil (e.g. in manufactured cakes and biscuits)
- Eat more chicken and any non-salted fish, particularly oily fish
- Eat more fresh fruit and vegetables (more than 5 servings/day)
- Use a monounsaturated fat (e.g. olive oil or rapeseed oil) or, if not available, a polyunsaturated fat (e.g. sunflower or corn oil)

Benefits of lowering cholesterol. There are now many trials showing the benefits of lowering cholesterol both in primary and secondary prevention of cardiovascular disease, some of which have included individuals with high blood pressure.

The ASCOT study included a double-blind arm, comparing atorvastatin, 10 mg, with placebo in approximately 10 000 individuals being treated for raised blood pressure. Total cholesterol had to be less than 6.5 mmol/L. The results showed a reduction in strokes and heart attacks of approximately one-third with the statin therapy (Figure 5.3). Importantly, the benefit was independent of the starting level of cholesterol.

The guidelines now recommend that any individual with high blood pressure who has signs of cardiovascular disease, a cholesterol level greater than 6.5 mmol/L or a cardiovascular risk of more than 20%, should definitely receive cholesterol-lowering therapy, usually a statin. Many healthcare professionals feel that if blood-pressure-lowering drugs are being given to prevent a stroke or heart attack, it makes sense to add a statin, as this approximately doubles the benefit. Consideration should perhaps be given to starting statin therapy in individuals on drug therapy for high blood pressure unless

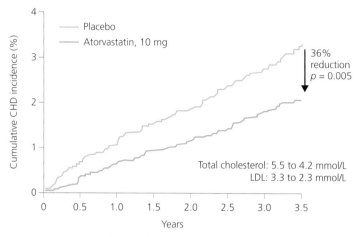

Figure 5.3 Comparison of statin therapy with placebo in the ASCOT study in patients with a starting cholesterol level < 6.5 mmol/L being treated for high blood pressure. Note the reduction in cholesterol levels. CHD, coronary heart disease; LDL, low-density lipoprotein. Adapted from Sever et al. 2003, with permission from Elsevier. Copyright © 2003.

there is a contraindication, particularly in men over 50 years of age or in women over 60 years of age, irrespective of cardiovascular risk.

Pharmacological treatment

The patient's blood pressure level will determine how quickly drug therapy is initiated. All those with mild-to-moderate hypertension should be given at least 3 months of non-pharmacological treatment, because blood pressure may fall to levels that do not require drug treatment in a large proportion of patients.

The four principal drug classes currently used in the treatment of high blood pressure are:
- diuretics
- calcium antagonists
- angiotensin-converting-enzyme (ACE) inhibitors
- angiotensin-receptor blockers (ARBs).

Ideally, patients should be tried on several classes as individuals have varying responses to different drugs and may experience different side effects. In reality, however, this may not be practical.

Multiple outcome trials measuring morbidity and mortality have been completed over the past 10 years comparing various drugs against one another as monotherapy. Other than for some expected differences (e.g. lesser efficacy of ACE inhibitors in black patients), all four classes of agent have provided similar degrees of protection against stroke and heart attack. However, the results of ASCOT show that this may not be the case as newer therapies provided better outcomes than did older ones. As will be noted, the presence of comorbidities, such as heart failure or nephropathy, provides compelling indications for which type of agent to use.

Diuretics. There are three major groups of diuretics:
- thiazides (e.g. hydrochlorothiazide, bendroflumethiazide) and many other related thiazide or allied drugs (e.g. chlortalidone, indapamide)
- loop diuretics (e.g. furosemide, bumetanide, torasemide)
- potassium-sparing diuretics (e.g. amiloride, triamterene, spironolactone, eplerenone).

These agents, particularly thiazides, continue to have a central role in the management of hypertension. The benefits of thiazide diuretics have been demonstrated in outcome trials, particularly in the elderly.

Thiazide diuretics act by inhibiting tubular sodium and chloride resorption, thereby causing loss of sodium chloride and a decrease in extracellular volume, resulting in a fall in blood pressure. This fall in blood pressure is, in part, blocked by a compensatory increase in renin release and, therefore, a rise in angiotensin II. As a result, diuretics are more effective on their own in patients who have a less reactive renin system (e.g. the elderly and black patients).

There is a dose response, but low doses of thiazides (e.g. hydrochlorothiazide, 12.5 mg, or bendroflumethiazide, 1.25 mg) are almost as effective as higher doses, and have the advantage of being much better tolerated and having fewer metabolic effects (e.g. hypokalemia). Thiazides have a markedly additive effect to drugs that inhibit the renin system, that is, ACE inhibitors and ARBs.

In general, thiazide diuretics are well tolerated, but importantly they may cause impotence in men, particularly at high dosages.

Thiazide diuretics can also cause a reduction in plasma potassium. This effect depends on the dose of the thiazide and the salt intake; the higher the salt intake, the greater the fall in plasma potassium. A fall in potassium may make patients more predisposed to ventricular arrhythmias and sudden death. Plasma potassium should be checked, and any fall minimized by restricting salt intake, using a potassium-sparing agent in combination with a thiazide, or by adding an ACE inhibitor or ARB.

Occasionally, thiazide diuretics will increase blood sugar and precipitate diabetes, particularly if used in combination with a β-blocker. They will also increase uric acid levels and occasionally cause gout.

Loop diuretics block sodium resorption in the ascending loop of Henlé, but in general they have a shorter duration of action than thiazide diuretics. Unless they are taken several times a day (twice or, better, three times a day), they have little effect on sodium balance and, therefore, do not lower blood pressure, unless salt intake is very low.

Traditionally, loop diuretics have been given for more resistant hypertension. They are particularly useful in patients with sodium and water retention due to heart failure or renal impairment, and have a marked additive effect when used in combination with thiazides.

Potassium-sparing diuretics act on the distal tubule to reduce potassium excretion and increase sodium excretion, and combined with low-dose thiazides, they will prevent the fall in plasma potassium. In patients with primary aldosteronism, spironolactone – a direct antagonist of aldosterone – is useful, although it has some endocrine side effects; amiloride is a useful alternative. Each of these agents can very rarely cause potentially dangerous hyperkalemia in patients with impaired renal function, particularly if there is a sudden change in renal function (e.g. rejection of renal transplant). They should be used with caution when combined with an ACE inhibitor or ARB. Eplenerone is a newer aldosterone antagonist that is effective and appears to lack some of the endocrine side effects of spironolactone.

Calcium antagonists, also known as calcium-channel blockers, act by inhibiting the entry of calcium into vascular smooth muscle thus causing muscle relaxation and vasodilation. Although these drugs are described as one class, there are major differences between them, and they are usefully split further into:

- dihydropyridines (e.g. amlodipine, nifedipine etc.)
- verapamil
- diltiazem.

Dihydropyridines are probably the most potent vasodilators and have little effect on cardiac conduction or contractility. They also cause loss of sodium almost equal to that seen with a diuretic. On their own, these agents are particularly effective in older patients and black patients, and efficacy increases with rising initial blood pressure.

Nearly all of the older compounds are short acting, including the most widely used, nifedipine, but this has now been produced in a slow-release preparation that acts over 24 hours (nifedipine gastro-intestinal therapeutic system; GITS). Amlodipine, the only naturally long-acting dihydropyridine calcium antagonist, has a half-life of 3 days and can be given once a day, or indeed every other day. It has a slower onset of action, only affecting blood pressure after 2–3 days.

When nifedipine GITS or amlodipine is given, fewer vasodilating side effects are seen (e.g. headache, flushing), although these do occur occasionally. All dihydropyridines can cause ankle edema, particularly in women, as a result of changes in local capillary hemodynamics (i.e. it is not due to sodium and water retention). This edema can be minimized by concomitant use of an ACE inhibitor or a reduction in dose. Nocturia in men is a common side effect and gingival hyperplasia may occur.

Verapamil is as effective at lowering blood pressure as the dihydropyridines. It slows the heart rate and causes some reduction in cardiac contractility. It is a short-acting drug, but various slow-release formulations are available, which can be given once or twice a day. It is important to check that the slow-release preparation lasts for the full 24 hours.

Verapamil is not associated, on the whole, with vasodilating side effects or edema, but does cause constipation. However, this can generally be overcome by eating a higher fiber fruit and vegetable diet or by consuming additional bran. Care should be taken with verapamil in patients with heart failure. In general use, it should not be combined with a β-blocker in view of the profound reduction in heart rate that can occur in some patients.

Diltiazem can also be used in the treatment of high blood pressure. Like verapamil it is short acting and needs to be given in a slow-release preparation, many of which do not last for the full 24 hours. Like verapamil it does have some mild negative chronotropic and inotropic effects. A study comparing a diltiazem-based regimen with a diuretic-based regimen showed an equal effect on cardiovascular outcome. The side effects observed with diltiazem lie between those of verapamil and the dihydropyridines.

ACE inhibitors were specifically developed to block the enzyme that converts angiotensin I to angiotensin II and thereby cause a fall in angiotensin II levels. Angiotensin II is the most powerful arteriolar vasoconstrictor in the body, and also has an effect on sodium and water retention both directly and through aldosterone. In addition, it stimulates the sympathetic nervous system both peripherally and centrally. Not surprisingly, therefore, drugs that block this system are effective in lowering blood pressure.

Because of their mode of action, they are particularly effective when combined with methods that increase angiotensin II (i.e. salt restriction, diuretics, calcium antagonists).

ACE inhibitors are generally well tolerated, and most patients feel well on them. There are, however, important side effects.

- A dry cough has been noted in up to 15% of those taking ACE inhibitors. It varies from the mildest upper respiratory tract irritation to spasms of severe coughing.
- Very rarely, ACE inhibitors cause angioedema that is often unrecognized and results in sudden swelling around the mouth and face. If this occurs, the drug should be stopped immediately as the angioedema could affect the larynx, with serious

consequences. Angioedema occurs with a higher incidence in black individuals.

- ACE inhibitors may cause a reduction in glomerular filtration rate in patients with critical renal artery stenosis. If there is only one functioning kidney or bilateral renovascular stenosis, this will cause a deterioration in kidney function. This particularly occurs if the individual is sodium and water depleted (e.g. as a result of severe food poisoning). It is important, therefore, in patients who are at risk of renal artery stenosis, and ideally in all patients, that renal function is checked before and after starting an ACE inhibitor.
- ACE inhibitors are contraindicated in pregnancy.

Therapy based on ACE inhibitors has been shown to be equal in efficacy to therapy based on a diuretic. In addition, ACE inhibitors have been shown to reduce mortality and morbidity in patients with heart failure and in patients with impairment of left ventricular function following myocardial infarction. At the same time, there is considerable evidence that ACE inhibitors delay the rate of deterioration of renal function in patients with diabetic nephropathy and in those with renal impairment due to intrinsic renal disease.

There are a number of ACE inhibitors available (Table 5.4). The only obvious differences between them are their durations of action and whether they need to be converted from an inactive metabolite. Many need to be given twice a day to maintain 24-hour control of blood pressure (e.g. enalapril, lisinopril, ramipril). It may be better to use a longer-acting ACE inhibitor such as perindopril or trandolapril. On their own, ACE inhibitors are less effective in the

TABLE 5.4

ACE inhibitors in clinical use in the UK and/or USA

• Captopril	• Imidapril	• Quinapril
• Cilazapril	• Lisinopril	• Ramipril
• Enalapril	• Moexipril	• Trandolapril
• Fosinopril	• Perindopril	

TABLE 5.5

Angiotensin-receptor blockers in clinical use in the UK and/or USA

• Candesartan	• Losartan	• Telmisartan
• Eprosartan	• Olmesartan	• Valsartan
• Irbesartan		

elderly and in black patients. However, when combined with salt restriction, diuretics or calcium antagonists, they are equally effective in all patients.

Angiotensin-receptor blockers specifically block angiotensin II from binding to its AT1 receptors (Table 5.5). These receptors mediate all the physiological effects of angiotensin and are therefore an effective way of blocking the effects of angiotensin II and causing a fall in blood pressure.

These drugs are remarkably free from side effects and, in particular, do not cause the cough associated with ACE inhibitors. Like ACE inhibitors, ARBs should be used with caution in patients with renal artery stenosis and are contraindicated in pregnancy. They give good blood pressure control when taken once a day. ARBs, like ACE inhibitors, are additive to diuretics and calcium antagonists. The LIFE study showed a decrease in strokes and new-onset diabetes in patients receiving losartan compared with atenolol. In diabetic renal disease, a reduction in the rate of deterioration in renal function has also been demonstrated with ARB therapy.

General principles of drug treatment

Treatment should be tailored to the individual's needs (Table 5.6). Hypertension is usually asymptomatic and treatment will need to be continued for a long time, usually for life. Thus, adverse events related to drug treatment may have a substantial impact on quality of life. If first-line treatment does not control blood pressure, two options should be considered:

• switching to another first-line agent
• adding a second drug.

The first option is appropriate if the patient experiences side effects with the first drug or if there has been no fall in blood pressure. However, if blood pressure is lowered but not controlled, it may be better to add a second drug.

Combination therapy may permit the use of lower doses, thus reducing the risk of adverse events. Combination treatment should involve drugs that have complementary mechanisms of action and, hence, additive effects on blood pressure (e.g. diuretics and/or salt restriction with an ACE inhibitor or ARB).

Drug combinations that have additive effects on blood pressure are shown in Figure 5.4. This simple additive treatment regimen is based on an arbitrary age cut-off, that is, younger non-black individuals (under 55 years of age) generally respond better to inhibition of the renin-angiotensin system with an ACE inhibitor or ARB, whereas older individuals (55 years and older) respond better to a calcium antagonist or diuretic. If blood pressure is not controlled, then one of the opposite drugs is added. If, with these

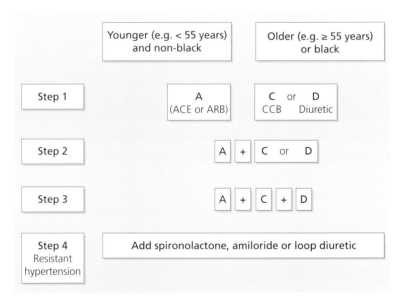

Figure 5.4 Drug combinations with additive effects on blood pressure.
A, angiotensin-converting-enzyme (ACE) inhibitor or angiotensin-receptor blocker (ARB); C, calcium antagonist (CCB, calcium-channel blocker); D, thiazide diuretic.

TABLE 5.6

Compelling and possible indications, contraindications and cautions for the four major classes of antihypertensive drug

Class of drug	Compelling indications	Possible indications
Thiazides	Elderly Heart failure Recurrent stroke prevention	Chronic renal disease Diabetes
Calcium antagonists (dihydropyridine)	Elderly isolated systolic hypertension	Angina PVD
Calcium antagonists (rate-limiting)	Angina	Myocardial infarction
ACE inhibitors	Heart failure Left ventricular dysfunction Type 1 diabetic nephropathy	Chronic renal disease Type 2 diabetic nephropathy
Angiotensin-receptor blockers	ACE-inhibitor-induced cough Type 2 diabetic nephropathy	Heart failure Intolerance of other antihypertensive drugs

ACE, angiotensin-converting-enzyme; PVD, peripheral vascular disease.
*ACE inhibitors may be beneficial in chronic renal failure but should only be used with caution, close supervision and specialist advice when there is established and significant renal impairment.

two drugs, blood pressure is still not controlled then either the diuretic or calcium antagonist is added, whichever has not been used. There is no advantage in adding an ACE inhibitor to an ARB, particularly if a reasonable dose of either drug is given. Fourth-line therapy is very much a matter of choice and experience, that is, based on little clinical trial evidence. Our own view is that it is more effective to add a distally acting diuretic such as amiloride or spironolactone (note you will need to check the plasma potassium) or a loop diuretic such as frusemide. Others would add α-blockers such as doxazosin or centrally acting drugs such as monodixine. Either way, these individuals should be referred to a specialist in high blood pressure as there is likely to be an underlying cause.

Possible contraindications	Compelling contraindications
Dyslipidemia	Gout
Combination with β-blockade	Heart block
	Heart failure
Renal impairment*	Pregnancy
PVD†	Bilateral renovascular disease
PVD†	Pregnancy
	Bilateral renovascular disease

†Caution should be exercised with ACE inhibitors and angiotensin-receptor blockers in PVD because of association with renovascular disease.

Other drugs used in the treatment of hypertension

β-blockers were first introduced in the 1960s and were widely used in the 1970s and 1980s. Recent trial evidence (see page 46) suggests that they are less effective than other drugs, particularly in reducing strokes and left ventricular hypertrophy, and cause more new-onset diabetes, particularly in combination with a diuretic. β-blockers also have obvious side effects, leading to a reduction in peripheral blood flow and worsening of Raynaud's syndrome or claudication. They may cause bronchoconstriction and aggravate asthma, and cause a reduction in exercise tolerance. They also have central nervous system side effects, which present as reduced mental agility and enjoyment of life for many patients. These subtle effects

> **Key points – how to treat**
>
> - Treatment of hypertension should always begin and continue with appropriate changes in lifestyle.
> - Moderate dietary sodium reduction provides multiple benefits and is relatively easy to achieve.
> - The choice of initial drug therapy may logically be based upon patients' age and race.
> - A combination of drugs will usually be needed to accomplish adequate control.
> - Choices should always include those drugs for which compelling indications exist.

need to be looked for, as individuals may not be aware of them, and only those living with the individual may have noticed these changes.

β-blockers are effective in relieving angina and have been shown to reduce mortality from heart failure and post-myocardial infarction. Many physicians would now feel that β-blockers' only indication for high blood pressure is in patients for whom treatment is indicated for these reasons.

Large numbers of individuals, particularly in the UK, have been on β-blockers for many years and with good control of blood pressure. Should these individuals have their therapy changed? The decision should be taken in consultation with the individual. Clearly, it is important, if treatment is changed (preferably to either an ACE inhibitor or ARB), to maintain good control of blood pressure. If there is any evidence or suggestion of underlying ischemic heart disease, the β-blocker should be continued; if withdrawn, it should be done gradually.

Alpha-blockers were developed predominantly to relieve the symptoms of prostatic hypertrophy, for which they can be effective. They do lower blood pressure and, in particular, may cause postural drops in blood pressure. Doxazosin is quite widely used in some countries for the treatment of high blood pressure. However, in the ALLHAT study (see page 44), the doxazosin arm was stopped due to an increase in the number of patients with heart failure and because of less effective control of blood pressure. α-blockers can be used as fourth-line therapy if the four major classes of drugs fail to control blood pressure, and in men with prostatic symptoms that are relieved by α-blockers, who also have high blood pressure. In women, they commonly cause urinary incontinence and should not be used.

Centrally acting drugs. These include methyldopa, clonidine and moxonidine. These drugs are no longer widely used because of their side effects. Methyldopa still has a role in pregnancy-induced hypertension (see page 75).

Key references

ALLHAT Collaborative Research Group. Major outcomes in high-risk hypertensive patients randomized to angiotensin-converting enzyme inhibitor or calcium channel blocker vs diuretic. The Antihypertensive and Lipid-Lowering treatment to prevent Heart Attack Trial (ALLHAT). *JAMA* 2002;288:2981–97.

Antonios TFT, MacGregor GA. Salt – more adverse effects. *Lancet* 1996;348:250–1.

Appel LJ, Moore TJ, Obarzanek E et al. A clinical trial of the effects of dietary patterns on blood pressure. *N Engl J Med* 1997;336:1117–24.

Bazzano LA, He J, Ogden LG et al. Dietary potassium intake and risk of stroke in US men and women. National Health and Nutrition Examination Survey I: epidemiologic follow-up study. *Stroke* 2001;32: 1473–80.

Brown MJ, Cruickshank JK, Dominiczak AF et al. Better blood pressure control: how to combine drugs. *J Hum Hypertens* 2003;17: 81–6.

Copeland SR, Mills MC, Lerner JL et al. Hemodynamic effects of aerobic vs resistance exercise. *J Hum Hypertens* 1996;10:747–53.

Elliott HL, Elawad M, Wilkinson R, Singh SP. Persistence of antihypertensive efficacy after missed doses: comparison of amlodipine and nifedipine gastrointestinal therapeutic system. *J Hypertens* 2002;20:333–8.

Forette F, Seux ML, Staessen JA et al. The prevention of dementia with hypertensive treatment. *Arch Intern Med* 2002;162:2046–52.

Hansson L, Zanchetti A, Carruthers SG et al. Effects of intensive blood-pressure lowering and low-dose aspirin in patients with hypertension: principal results of the Hypertension Optimal Treatment randomised trial. *Lancet* 1998;351:1755–62.

He FJ, MacGregor GA. How far should salt intake be reduced? *Hypertension* 2003;42:1093–99.

Knowler WC, Barrett-Connor E, Fowler SE et al. Reduction in the incidence of type 2 diabetes with lifestyle intervention or metformin. *N Engl J Med* 2002;346:393–403.

Malhotra A, White DP. Obstructive sleep apnoea. *Lancet* 2002;360: 237–45.

Messerli FH, Grossman E, Goldbourt U. Are beta-blockers efficacious as first-line therapy for hypertension in the elderly? A systematic review. *JAMA* 1998;279:1903–7.

Mukamal KJ, Kuller LH, Fitzpatrick AL et al. Prospective study of alcohol consumption and risk of dementia in older adults. *JAMA* 2003;289: 1405–13.

Sareli P, Radevski IV, Valtchanova ZP et al. Efficacy of different drug classes used to initiate antihypertensive treatment in black subjects. *Arch Intern Med* 2001;161:965–71.

Sever PS, Dahlof B, Poulter NR et al. Prevention of coronary and stroke events with atorvastatin in hypertensive patients who have lower-than-average cholesterol concentrations, in the ASCOT-LLA: a multicentre randomised controlled trial. *Lancet* 2003;361:1149–58.

Steptoe A, Perkins-Porras L, McKay C et al. Behavioural counselling to increase consumption of fruit and vegetables in low income adults: randomised trial. *BMJ* 2003;326: 855–60.

Tuomilehto J, Jousilahti P, Rastenyte D et al. Urinary sodium excretion and cardiovascular mortality in Finland: a prospective study. *Lancet* 2001;357:848–51.

Weinberger MH, Roniker B, Krause SL, Weiss R. Eplerenone, a selective aldosterone blocker, in mild-to-moderate hypertension. *Am J Hypertens* 2002;15:709–16.

Whelton PK, He J, Appel LJ et al. Primary prevention of hypertension: clinical and public health advisory from the National High Blood Pressure Education Program. *JAMA* 2002;288:1882–8.

Williams B. Drug treatment of hypertension. *BMJ* 2003;326:61–2.

Wing LMH, Reid CM, Ryan P et al. A comparison of outcomes with angiotensin-converting-enzyme inhibitors and diuretics for hypertension in the elderly. *N Engl J Med* 2003;348:583–92.

Yusuf S, Sleight P, Pogue J et al. The HOPE Study Investigators. Effects of an angiotensin-converting-enzyme inhibitor, ramipril, on cardiovascular events in high-risk patients. *N Engl J Med* 2000;342:145–53.

The investigation and management of hypertension requires particular attention in certain patient groups, notably:

- children
- pregnant women
- the elderly
- patients with diabetes.

Children

Although hypertension is rare in prepubertal children, it is becoming more common as obesity becomes more widespread. If a prepubertal child has a blood pressure level that would be considered raised in an adult, it is almost always associated with an underlying disease (e.g. renal or adrenal). The diagnosis is complicated by difficulties in measuring blood pressure in children; conventional sphygmomanometry is not feasible for patients under 5 years old, and careful attention must be paid to cuff size for older children (see Table 3.1, page 31). It is also necessary to measure leg blood pressure in children with high arm blood pressure, to exclude the possibility of coarctation of the aorta.

A child's blood pressure increases during the first 6 weeks of life, and then remains almost constant until the age of 5, after which pressures increase gradually to adult levels. Normal blood pressure in children varies according to age, sex and height. Hypertension in children has recently been defined as average systolic pressure and/or diastolic pressure from three or more measurements that is greater than or equal to the 95th percentile for age, sex and height. In the USA, the National High Blood Pressure Education Program Working Group on High Blood Pressure in Children and Adolescents has published data on normal blood pressure in children (Table 6.1), along with recommendations for diagnosis, evaluation and treatment of hypertension.

TABLE 6.1

95th percentile of blood pressure by age, sex and height in children

| Age (years) | Systolic/diastolic blood pressure (mmHg) | | | |
| | 50th percentile for height | | 75th percentile for height | |
	Boys	Girls	Boys	Girls
1	103/56	104/58	104/57	105/59
6	114/74	111/74	115/75	113/74
12	123/81	123/80	125/82	124/81
17	136/87	129/84	138/87	130/85

Adapted from data available at
http://pediatrics.aappublications.org/cgi/reprint/114/2/S2/555.pdf

Children should have their blood pressure measured by the age of 5, initially to identify those with high blood pressure. Such children must be referred to a pediatrician with an interest in high blood pressure, as the hypertension is very likely to have an underlying cause.

Non-pharmacological advice should be given for children in the upper quartile of blood pressures, in particular:
• reduce salt intake
• increase potassium intake
• lose weight (as most of these children are overweight).
The principles of antihypertensive treatment for children are similar to those in adults, and the first-line drugs used in adults are also suitable, in general, for children, though doses must be corrected for the child's age and weight.

Pregnancy
Hypertension during pregnancy can take several forms (Table 6.2).

Essential hypertension. Approximately 5% of young women have essential hypertension, and this figure increases to about 10% in

TABLE 6.2

Classification of hypertension during pregnancy

- Pre-existing hypertension
  - essential
  - secondary
- Pregnancy-induced or gestational hypertension
- Pre-eclampsia

women in their late 30s and early 40s. This elevated blood pressure may decrease during the first trimester of pregnancy, but may subsequently return to pre-conception levels.

Well-managed essential hypertension in pregnancy is not associated with a poor prognosis for the mother or fetus. However, if blood pressure measurements before pregnancy are not available, it is difficult to distinguish this condition from pregnancy-induced hypertension (PIH), which is often treated inappropriately as a result.

Secondary hypertension due to a pheochromocytoma can lead to both maternal and fetal death. Hypertension associated with renal disease may be associated with a poor prognosis for the fetus, and may accelerate the rate of deterioration in renal function in the mother.

Pregnancy-induced hypertension occurs in women who are normotensive before and after pregnancy. This condition has been arbitrarily defined as a single diastolic pressure (phase V) of at least 110 mmHg, or at least two measurements of 90 mmHg or more 4 hours apart, occurring after the 20th week of pregnancy, provided blood pressure was normal previously. It occurs in up to 25% of first pregnancies and 10% of subsequent pregnancies. The immediate prognosis is good provided that pre-eclampsia does not develop. However, women who have had hypertension in pregnancy have an increased risk of later developing raised blood pressure and stroke.

Pre-eclampsia is characterized by a raised blood pressure, edema and proteinuria (above 300 mg/L), occurring after the 20th week of pregnancy. Pre-eclampsia is a major cause of fetal growth retardation and death and, if untreated, can progress to eclampsia, which is associated with high maternal and fetal mortality. Pre-eclampsia occurs in about 5% of first pregnancies; the prevalence decreases in subsequent pregnancies. Women who develop pre-eclampsia have a long-term risk of developing persistent hypertension and cardiovascular disease.

Diagnosis and management. Blood pressure should be measured at least twice a month during the first two trimesters. The technique should be the same as in other patients (see Chapter 3). Diastolic pressure may be difficult to measure, as some sounds may be heard even at very low pressures. In general, the fifth Korotkoff sound should be recorded as diastolic blood pressure.

Women with a blood pressure of 140/90 mmHg or more at their first antenatal clinic visit are likely to have pre-existing essential or secondary hypertension. Such women should, if possible, be referred to a joint antenatal–hypertension clinic. Women with mild hypertension (150/100 mmHg or below) before the 20th week of pregnancy should not be treated with drugs. Treatment after the 20th week of pregnancy depends on the cause of hypertension.

- Women with mild PIH (blood pressure between 140/90 and 160/110 mmHg) can usually be managed at home, initially by reduction of physical activity; however, complete bedrest is not recommended and may actually be harmful. If blood pressure remains elevated, treatment with the centrally acting α-agonist methyldopa or labetalol can be started.
- Pre-eclampsia requires immediate hospital admission for assessment and treatment. Blood pressure should be controlled as above. Magnesium sulfate should be used if eclampsia threatens.

Contraindications. Certain groups of antihypertensive drugs are contraindicated during pregnancy. In particular, the addition of a thiazide diuretic may worsen plasma volume and uteroplacental blood flow in women with pre-eclampsia, and angiotensin-converting-enzyme (ACE) inhibitors and angiotensin-receptor blockers (ARBs) have been shown to be associated with congenital abnormalities, fetal retardation and intrauterine death. In addition, there is insufficient experience with calcium antagonists during pregnancy to recommend their use except where more old-fashioned drugs fail to control blood pressure. β-blockers can cause growth retardation in the first trimester.

Elderly patients

As described in Chapter 4, there is strong evidence that elderly patients benefit from antihypertensive treatment. Drug treatment should be given if systolic pressure is consistently above 140 mmHg despite non-pharmacological measures.

Calcium antagonists and diuretics are more effective as first-line agents than ACE inhibitors or ARBs. Drug doses may need to be adjusted for declining renal or liver function. It may be particularly important with the diuretics to prevent any fall in potassium levels, as older patients usually have a low potassium intake. Adding a distally acting diuretic, such as amiloride or triamterene, to the thiazide diuretic may be beneficial. It is also important to look for postural drops in blood pressure (i.e. measure standing blood pressure), which can lead to falls and hip fractures.

Patients with diabetes

Hypertension occurs in at least 30% of patients with type 1 diabetes mellitus and in the majority of patients with type 2 diabetes mellitus. Nephropathy develops in around 40% of patients with type 1 diabetes and is usually accompanied by hypertension. The majority of diabetic patients die from premature vascular disease, and it is vital to control their blood lipid levels and blood pressure.

Patients with diabetes have a poor prognosis once hypertension has developed, and thus it is recommended that treatment be started at lower blood pressure levels than those in the non-diabetic population. Since those with type 2 diabetes are usually overweight,

> **Key points – special patient groups**
>
> - As a result of increasing obesity, hypertension is being seen in more children.
> - Hypertension during pregnancy must be recognized early and carefully managed.
> - Treatment of the growing number of elderly hypertensives provides excellent protection against stroke.
> - Diabetic patients have a high prevalence of hypertension, which must be intensively treated.

attention to diet and physical activity is critical. Pharmacological treatment is recommended if systolic pressure is above 130 mmHg or diastolic blood pressure is above 80 mmHg.

ACE inhibitors and ARBs may possibly have advantages over other classes of agent, as they have been shown to:
- reduce the development of proteinuria in diabetics with microalbuminuria
- reduce urinary albumin excretion in patients with established proteinuria
- delay the progression of diabetic renal disease.

Drug choices. Most diabetics will require combination therapy to control blood pressure. There is some evidence to suggest that ACE inhibitors or ARBs may slow down the rate of deterioration in renal function, and all diabetics who are being treated for high blood pressure should either include an ACE inhibitor or ARB in their treatment regimen.

Calcium antagonists and diuretics are additive to these drugs and should be added in the same way as in essential hypertension (see pages 67–8). If possible, blood pressure should be lowered to below 130/80 mmHg for maximum benefit. All patients with type 2 diabetes must be treated with a statin to lower total cholesterol and low-density lipoprotein (LDL) cholesterol.

Key references

American Academy of Pediatrics.
The Fourth Report on the Diagnosis,
Evaluation, and Treatment of High
Blood Pressure in Children and
Adolescents. National High Blood
Pressure Education Program Working
Group on High Blood Pressure in
Children and Adolescents. *Pediatrics*
2004;114:555–76.
http://pediatrics.aappublications.org/
cgi/reprint/114/2/S2/555.pdf

Bakris GL, Williams M, Dworkin L
et al. for the National Kidney
Foundation Hypertension and
Diabetes Executive Committees
Working Group. Preserving renal
function in adults with hypertension
and diabetes: a consensus approach.
Am J Kidney Dis 2000;36:646–61.

Bath P, Chalmers J, Powers W et al.
International Society of Hypertension
(ISH): statement on the management
of blood pressure in acute stroke.
J Hypertens 2003;21:665–72.

Flynn JT. Pharmacologic
management of childhood
hypertension: current status, future
challenges. *Am J Hypertens* 2002;
15:30S–33S.

Gaede P, Vedel P, Larsen N et al.
Multifactorial intervention and
cardiovascular disease in patients
with type 2 diabetes. *N Engl J Med*
2003;348:383–93.

Ingelfinger JR. Pediatric antecedents
of adult cardiovascular disease –
awareness and intervention.
N Engl J Med 2004;350:2123–6.

Nakao N, Yoshimura A, Morita H
et al. Combination treatment of
angiotensin-II receptor blocker and
angiotensin-converting-enzyme
inhibitor in non-diabetic renal disease
(COOPERATE): a randomised
controlled trial. *Lancet* 2003;361:
117–24.

Remuzzi G, Schieppati A, Ruggenenti
P. Clinical practice. Nephropathy in
patients with type 2 diabetes. *N Engl
J Med* 2002;346:1145–51.

Staessen JA, Gasowski J, Wang JG
et al. Risks of untreated and treated
isolated systolic hypertension in the
elderly: meta-analysis of outcome
trials. *Lancet* 2000;355:865–72.

Tuomilehto J, Rastenyte D,
Birkenhager WH et al.; Systolic
Hypertension in Europe Trial
Investigators. Effects of calcium-
channel blockade in older patients
with diabetes and systolic
hypertension. *N Engl J Med*
1999;340:677–84.

UK Prospective Diabetes Study
Group. Tight blood pressure control
and risk of macrovascular and
microvascular complications in
type 2 diabetes: UKPDS 38. *BMJ*
1998;317:703–13.

Wilson BJ, Watson MS, Prescott GJ
et al. Hypertensive diseases of
pregnancy and risk of hypertension
and stroke in later life: results from
cohort study. *BMJ* 2003;326:845–51.

Wright JT Jr, Bakris G, Greene T et al. Effect of blood pressure lowering and antihypertensive drug class on progression of hypertensive kidney disease: results from the AASK trial. *JAMA* 2002;288: 2421–31.

Zanchetti A, Ruilope LM. Antihypertensive treatment in patients with type-2 diabetes mellitus: what guidance from recent controlled randomized trials? *J Hypertens* 2002;20:2099–110.

Despite the clear benefits of lowering raised blood pressure, a large number of individuals do not receive adequate treatment. In much of the world, the so-called 'rule of halves' applies (Figure 7.1), and only 12.5% of people with hypertension receive adequate treatment. Recent studies show that in many European countries, fewer than 20% of patients are controlled to a target level of 140/90 mmHg; in the USA, the corresponding figure is about 30%. In the UK alone, approximately 60 000 deaths from strokes and heart attacks would be prevented if all individuals who needed treatment were controlled to 140/90 mmHg.

Reasons for this unsatisfactory situation include failure to measure blood pressure routinely, lack of appreciation of the risks associated with high blood pressure, poor patient compliance, and treatment with too few drugs or illogical combinations of drugs.

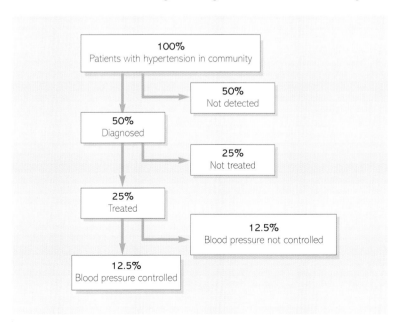

Figure 7.1 Rule of halves.

These problems can be overcome by making efforts to identify those individuals with hypertension and closely monitoring their long-term treatment. This requires screening large numbers of people – blood pressure should be measured at every opportunity. Everyone should know what their blood pressure is, just as they are aware of their height and weight. The individual should be given the knowledge to put themselves in charge.

Routine measurement

Most hypertensive patients are asymptomatic, so that hypertension can be diagnosed only by routine measurement of blood pressure. Primary care physicians have a leading role to play in screening for hypertension because they are the patient's first point of contact with the healthcare system in most countries.

Associated risks

There appears to be a widespread misconception that mild hypertension is a less important health problem than severe hypertension. Severe hypertension is, indeed, a major cause of premature death, but it is relatively rare. In contrast, mild hypertension is common, affecting about 20% of the middle-aged population and well over 50% of people over 70 years of age. Thus, although mild hypertension is associated with a lower absolute risk than severe hypertension, prevention and treatment of this condition could substantially reduce cardiovascular morbidity and mortality because of the very large number of people affected.

Patient compliance

Compliance with treatment is often poor in patients with hypertension. In some cases, this is due to side effects of drug treatment that can impair patients' quality of life. Furthermore, because of the usually asymptomatic nature of hypertension, patients may not perceive any benefit from treatment and thus be unwilling to continue taking medication in the long term. The importance of effective treatment therefore needs to be carefully explained to all patients.

Screening for hypertension

Opportunistic screening. It is estimated that 70–80% of the population will visit their primary care physician at least once during a 3-year period. Hence, measuring blood pressure at these visits (opportunistic screening) provides a means of screening the population for hypertension. Patients should have their blood pressures checked if they have not consulted their doctor within the previous 12 months, and subsequent management should be based on the pressure found.

Selective screening. A strong case can be made for screening those patients known to have a high risk of hypertension or hypertensive complications (Table 7.1).

The role of the specialist

Until recently, patients with hypertension were thought to be adequately managed in the primary care setting, with less than 10% being referred to a specialist. Those referred included:

- patients in whom underlying disease was suspected as a cause of hypertension
- patients with evidence of end organ damage, such as proteinuria or renal failure
- patients under the age of 40 years with any degree of hypertension
- patients in whom blood pressure was not being controlled by adequate pharmacological and non-pharmacological therapy.

TABLE 7.1

Patients at high risk of hypertension suitable for selective screening

- Patients with a family history of hypertension, coronary heart disease or stroke
- Patients with previous vascular complications of hypertension
- Patients with diabetes
- Patients with other systemic diseases (including renal disease and peripheral vascular disease)

However, given that most patients with high blood pressure are not having their blood pressure controlled and many are started on drug treatment without proper assessment, it might be more appropriate if most patients were initially assessed and investigated by someone with a particular interest in high blood pressure. Once blood pressure is controlled, follow-up can be transferred back to the primary care physician and/or nurse, who should work in collaboration with the hypertension specialist to ensure that potentially avoidable strokes and heart attacks are prevented.

Many patients can now measure their own blood pressure at home, and most of the automatic electronic blood pressure machines are very accurate. Putting the patient in charge of controlling their own blood pressure, where appropriate, is likely to be the most effective management.

Improving control of hypertension

Non-pharmacological treatment. If properly explained, dietary advice can result in very effective lowering of blood pressure as well as a reduction in cardiovascular risk. Such measures require time, effort and the cooperation of whoever cooks in the household.

Pharmacological treatment. All drugs that lower blood pressure have well-known side effects. They also have more minor and subtle side effects that can have a major impact on the patient's life. It is important to address these, as they can be a significant and quite justifiable reason for non-compliance.

Most physicians use an inadequate number of drugs in combination. Most patients require at least two, and more than a third require three drugs to achieve a target of 140/90 mmHg. Often, illogical combinations are given – see Figure 5.4, page 67 for a simple, logical approach to combination therapy.

The nurse's role. Well-trained and motivated nurses are by far the best at giving dietary advice, seeking out the more subtle effects of drugs, and ensuring better compliance with both non-pharmacological and pharmacological treatments.

Resistant hypertension

Perhaps 10% of patients with hypertension will be resistant (i.e. their blood pressure remains above 140/90 mmHg despite treatment with three appropriate medications including a diuretic). The reasons are often multiple (Table 7.2), but when patients are carefully assessed, the causes can usually be identified and overcome.

TABLE 7.2

Causes of resistant hypertension

Inaccurate measurement of blood pressure

Volume overload and pseudotolerance

- Excess sodium intake
- Volume retention from kidney disease
- Inadequate diuretic therapy

Drug-induced/other causes

- Non-compliance with drug regimen
- Inadequate drug doses
- Inappropriate drug combinations
- Non-steroidal anti-inflammatory drugs (NSAIDs); cyclo-oxygenase (COX)-2 inhibitors
- Cocaine, amphetamines, other illicit drugs
- Sympathomimetics (decongestants, anorectics)
- Oral contraceptives
- Adrenal steroids
- Ciclosporin and tacrolimus
- Erythropoietin
- Licorice (including some chewing tobacco)
- Selected over-the-counter dietary supplements and medicines (e.g. ephedra/ma huang, bitter orange)

Associated conditions

- Obesity
- Excess alcohol intake

Identifiable secondary causes of hypertension (see pages 22–26)

Key points – uncontrolled hypertension

- The majority of hypertensives are not being adequately controlled and therefore remain at added risk for premature cardiovascular diseases.
- The asymptomatic nature of most hypertension makes it a difficult condition to control over the long term.
- Multiple techniques have been found to improve patient adherence to therapy.

Key references

Appel LJ, Moore TJ, Obarzanek E et al. A clinical trial of the effects of dietary patterns on blood pressure. DASH Collaborative Research Group. *N Engl J Med* 1997;336: 1117–24.

Blair SN, Kampert JB, Kohl HW 3rd et al. Influences of cardiorespiratory fitness and other precursors on cardiovascular disease and all-cause mortality in men and women. *JAMA* 1996;276:205–10.

Haynes RB, McDonald HP, Garg AX. Helping patients follow prescribed treatment: clinical applications. *JAMA* 2002;288:2880–3.

Lloyd-Jones DM, Evans JC, Larson MG, Levy D. Treatment and control of hypertension in the community: a prospective analysis *Hypertension* 2002;40:640–6.

Mansoor GA, Frishman WH. Comprehensive management of hypertensive emergencies and urgencies. *Heart Dis* 2002;4:358–71.

Marques-Vidal P, Tuomilehto J. Hypertension awareness, treatment and control in the community: is the 'rule of halves' still valid? *J Hum Hypertens* 1997;11:213–20.

Whelton PK, Appel LJ, Espeland MA et al. Sodium reduction and weight loss in the treatment of hypertension in older persons: a randomized controlled trial of nonpharmacologic interventions in the elderly (TONE). TONE Collaborative Research Group. *JAMA* 1998;279:839–46.

Useful addresses

UK

Blood Pressure Association
60 Cranmer Terrace
London SW17 0QS
Tel: +44 (0)20 8772 4994
www.bpassoc.org.uk

British Heart Foundation
14 Fitzhardinge Street
London W1H 6DH
Tel: +44 (0)20 7935 0185
Heart info line: 08450 70 80 70

British Hypertension Society
Administrative Officer
Clinical Sciences Building
Level 5
Leicester Royal Infirmary
PO Box 65
Leicester LE2 7LX
Tel: +44 (0)7717 467973
bhs@le.ac.uk
www.bhsoc.org

Consensus Action on Salt & Health (CASH)
Blood Pressure Unit
Department of Medicine
St George's Hospital Medical
School, London SW17 0RE
Tel: +44 (0)20 8266 6498
cash@sghms.ac.uk
www.hyp.ac.uk/cash

North America

American Heart Association
National Center
7272 Greenville Avenue
Dallas, TX 75231
Tel: 1 800 242 8721
www.americanheart.org

American Society of Hypertension
148 Madison Avenue
Fifth Floor
New York, NY 10016
Tel: +1 212 696 9099
Fax: +1 212 696 0711
ash@ash-us.org
www.ash-us.org

The Canadian Hypertension Society
info@hypertension.ca
www.hypertension.ca

National Institutes of Health
9000 Rockville Pike
Bethesda
Maryland 20892
Tel: +1 301 496 4000
nihinfo@od.nih.gov
www.nih.gov

International

European Society of
Hypertension
info@eshonline.org
www.eshonline.org

International Society of
Hypertension in Blacks
100 Auburn Avenue NE
Suite 401
Atlanta, GA 30303, USA
Tel: +1 404 880 0343
Fax: +1 404 880 0347
inforequest@ishib.org
www.ishib.org

Southern African Hypertension
Society
PO Box 122, River Club
South Africa, 2149
Tel: +27 11 706 4196
Fax: +27 11 706 4915
sahs@hypertension.org.za
www.hypertension.org.za

World Heart Federation
(including the International
Society of Hypertension)
5, avenue du Mail
1205 Geneva, Switzerland
Tel: +41 22 807 03 20
Fax: +41 22 807 03 39
admin@worldheart.org
www.worldheart.org

Index

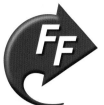

Imagine if every time you wanted to know something you knew where to look...

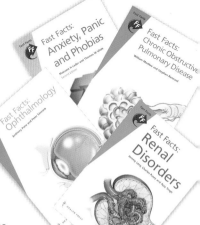

Over one million copies sold

- Written by world experts
- Concise and practical
- Up to date
- Designed for ease of reading and reference
- Copiously illustrated with useful photographs, diagrams and charts.

Our aim is to make *Fast Facts* the world's most respected medical handbook series. Feedback on how to make titles even more useful is always welcome (feedback@fastfacts.com).

More than 70 *Fast Facts* titles, including:

Anxiety, Panic and Phobias (second edition)
Asthma
Benign Gynecological Disease (second edition)
Benign Prostatic Hyperplasia (fifth edition)
Bipolar Disorder
Bladder Cancer
Bleeding Disorders
Brain Tumors
Breast Cancer (third edition)
Chronic Obstructive Pulmonary Disease
Colorectal Cancer (second edition)
Contraception (second edition)
Dementia
Depression (second edition)
Dyspepsia (second edition)
Eczema and Contact Dermatitis
Endometriosis (second edition)
Epilepsy (third edition)
Erectile Dysfunction (third edition)
Headaches (second edition)
Hyperlipidemia (third edition)

Inflammatory Bowel Disease (second edition)
Irritable Bowel Syndrome (second edition)
Menopause (second edition)
Minor Surgery
Multiple Sclerosis (second edition)
Ophthalmology
Osteoporosis (fourth edition)
Parkinson's Disease
Prostate Cancer (fourth edition)
Psoriasis (second edition)
Renal Disorders
Respiratory Tract Infection (second edition)
Rheumatoid Arthritis
Schizophrenia (second edition)
Sexual Dysfunction
Sexually Transmitted Infections
Skin Cancer
Smoking Cessation
Soft Tissue Rheumatology
Thyroid Disorders
Urinary Stones

Orders

To order via the website, or to find regional distributors, please go to www.fastfacts.com

For telephone orders, please call +44 (0)1752 202301 (Europe), 1 800 247 6553 (USA, toll free) or +1 419 281 1802 (Americas)